12.99

WB20
NOR

Evidence-Based
Medicine
in Sherlock Holmes' Footsteps

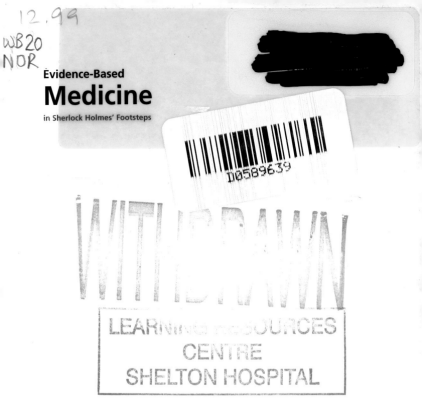

Evidence-Based
Medicine
in Sherlock Holmes' Footsteps

Jorgen Nordenstrom, MD, PhD

Professor of Surgery
Karolinska University Hospital
Karolinska Institutet
Sweden

Blackwell
Publishing

© 2007 Jörgen Nordenström
Published by Blackwell Publishing Ltd
Blackwell Publishing, Inc., 350 Main Street, Malden, MA 02148 5020, USA
Blackwell Publishing Ltd, 9600 Garsington Road, Oxford OX4 2DQ, UK
Blackwell Publishing Asia Pty Ltd, 550 Swanston Street, Carlton, Victoria 3053, Australia

First published 2007

1 2007

Originally published in Swedish by Karolinska University Press, Stockholm, Sweden

Library of Congress Cataloging-in-Publication Data
Nordenström, Jörgen.
  [Evidensbaserad medicin i Sherlock Holmes fotspår. English]
  Evidence-based medicine in Sherlock Holmes' footsteps / Jörgen
Nordenström.
    p. ; cm.
  Includes bibliographical references and index.
  ISBN-13: 978-1-4051-5713-1 (alk. paper)
  ISBN-10: 1-4051-5713-5 (alk. paper)
  1. Evidence-based medicinevHandbooks, manuals, etc.   I. Title.
  [DNLM: 1. Evidence-Based Medicine–methods–Handbooks.
  WB 39 N832e 2007a]
R723.7.N67 2007
616–dc22   2000602167

A catalogue record for this title is available from the British Library

Set in 8.75/11 pts Minion by Charon Tec Ltd (A Macmillan Company), Chennai, India,
www.charontec.com
Printed and bound in Singapore by COS Printers Pte Ltd

Commissioning Editor: Martin Sugden
Editorial Assistant: Eleanor Bonnet
Development Editor: Hayley Salter
Text and cover designer: Sarah Dickinson

For further information on Blackwell Publishing, visit our website:
http://www.blackwellpublishing.com

Contents

Foreword, vi
Introduction, ix

STEP 1 Formulate an Answerable Question, 1

STEP 2 Information Search, 19

STEP 3 Review of Information and Critical Appraisal, 35

STEP 4 Employ the Results in Your Daily Practice, 69

Deduction, Analysis and Medicine, 75

References, 78

Summary of Information Sources and Search Engines, 79

Internet-Based Spreadsheets, 81

Sherlock Holmes References, 82

List of Illustrations, 83

Recommended EBM Literature, 84

Glossary, 85

Index, 89

Foreword

When I discuss EBM with patients or the public, they are always surprised to find this is not something that doctors are not already routinely doing. Surely medical decisions with such important consequences are informed by the best available research evidence? Patients may doubt a doctor's diagnostic or procedural skills, but they rarely question a doctor's ability to access knowledge. We know the reality is different. As Dr Nordenstrom points out:

"Today students and practitioners of medicine have a huge amount of information resources at their fingertips, yet many feel uncertain about how to find the right articles to read and even more uncertain about how to interpret scientific data."

I would hope that all health care students everywhere now get a grounding in the principles of evidence-based practice. However, I suspect that is still not so – many medical schools I know spend more time on the insertions of muscles or the Kreb's cycle than on the principles of using medical research at the bedside. And even when it is taught it can often be seen as boring. This lively little book makes EBM both appealing and simple. The appeal to detective work as an analogy and the intimate style make the reading very accessible. And yet, despite its informal style and brevity, it manages to convey many of the essentials of EBM. Students could read this in a single evening, and would be much better armed to find and appraise the research literature relevant to the care of patients.

I hope this short book will stimulate you to read more widely about EBM, but if not you will have gotten the essentials. I am sure you will remember the FIRE by PICO matrix and ask better questions and perform better searches. Of course, the book covers just the basic scales of EBM, and you will need to practice, experiment and improvise to embed these skills as part of your lifelong learning about medicine. And you may just hear Holmes leaning over your shoulder saying "Education never ends, Watson. It is a series of lessons with the greatest for the last."

Paul Glasziou
Professor of Evidence-Based Medicine
University of Oxford
May 2006

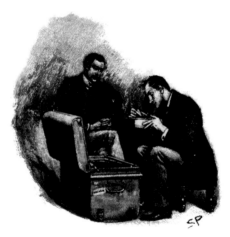

Any truth is better than indefinite doubt.
Sherlock Holmes in *The Yellow Face*.

Introduction

Evidence-based medicine (EBM) may be defined as "the integration of the best research evidence with clinical expertise and patient values" [1] and has been launched as a process by means of which advances in medical research may come into practical use so as to yield safer, better and more cost-effective health care. When the EBM concept first began to take hold critical voices were raised, claiming, among other things, that there was a risk of replacing clinical judgement with "cookbook medicine". But EBM has gradually defined itself and few people would now question its importance, which boils down to integrating clinical skills with the best available basic information obtainable based on systematically conducted clinical research.

Evidence is a fundamental concept for many practices (e.g. law and science) and professions (e.g. detectives and clinicians) and refers to the grounds for beliefs or judgements. In medicine, evidence is derived from many different activities including experimentation, observation and experience. The major contribution of EBM lies in the emphasis it places on a hierarchy of evidential reliability in which controlled experiments are accorded greater credibility than other types of evidence [2].

The application of EBM is based on three important principles. Firstly, high-quality health care rests on objective and clinically relevant information. Secondly, there is a hierarchy of evidence in which some types of evidence are stronger than others. Evidence as high up as possible in the hierarchy should be used and one must know the level at which a clinical decision is based. Thirdly, scientific data alone will not suffice for making clinical decisions and issuing recommendations; scientific information needs to be integrated with sound clinical judgement and the perceptions of patients as to the relative importance of different interventions and their results.

Today students and practitioners of medicine have a huge amount of information resources at their fingertips, yet many feel uncertain about how to find the right articles to read and even more uncertain about how to interpret scientific data. Additional problems include time shortages in the health services and a limited knowledge of the tools required (EBM portals, electronic library resources, etc.).

Information technology and the Internet have radically changed the way in which we produce data, store information and communicate. These developments have resulted in a democratization of the availability of information. More and more patients avail themselves of unsystematic and opinionated information, which makes new demands on all who work in the health care services. To guide and inform patients in the face of this torrent of information is a new and demanding challenge.

The need for EBM in health care work has gradually increased, partly owing to the fact that the medical knowledge pool is expanding exponentially. Consider the following:

- More than 15 million medical papers have been published.
- The number of medical journals is in excess of 5000.
- It has been estimated that only some 10–15% of what is published today will be of lasting scientific value.
- It has been estimated that half of today's medical knowledge base will be out-of-date, erroneous or irrelevant in 10 years.

The increased amount of information is usually characterized by such terms as a superabundance of information, a flood of information and a bibliometric explosion – expressions that lead one's thoughts to natural catastrophes and helplessness. Against this background, it is not surprising that the traditional sources of medical information function poorly:

- Textbooks quickly become outdated.
- As for journals, there are too many of them and they are often irrelevant to the immediate need.
- Experts may be wrong.

The increase in available information will continue and the ability to handle new information in general and new scientific data in particular will be a necessary component of the lifelong learning process. Skills in searching, evaluating and implementing are more important today than ever before. When should I change my processing routines? What new developments should be accepted? And which should be rejected?

The practice of EBM has similarities to detective work. In both instances, the initial stage consists in being confronted with a "case" in which certain events have preceded the current situation. In the detective work situation, a crime has been committed, there is a crime scene, there is a victim and a perpetrator, and events have occurred that need to be analysed. In the medical case, there is a patient who presents with certain symptoms and the task at hand is to make a diagnosis based on these symptoms and try to establish what preceded the onset of the illness. Both cases require a line of reasoning involving a temporal review and analysis, the so-called "backward reasoning", in order to establish causal relationships. This type of reasoning backwards in time constitutes an important principle in both health care work and problem-based learning (PBL). This pedagogic strategy was developed by Barrows towards the end of the 1970s at McMaster University in Canada, and it is no coincidence that the EBM concept was later developed at the same university.

Sherlock Holmes is the most famous private detective in history. His creator, Sir Arthur Conan Doyle, was a physician himself. The prototype of Sherlock Holmes was Dr Joseph Bell, one of Doyle's teachers at Edinburgh University. Doyle has reported how Bell usually tried to diagnose his patients at the very first consultation, even before they had uttered a single word. He is said to have been able to recount the symptoms of his patients, give an account of their medical history and relate details of their daily life with an amazing degree of accuracy. Sherlock Holmes' constant companion, Dr Watson, was a practising physician and Doyle's alter ego. Thus the two detectives' technique and *modus operandi* have, in part, a medical background. Conan Doyle once stated, "I thought I would try my hand at writing a story where the hero would treat crime as Dr Bell treated disease." According to legend, Sherlock Holmes was born on 6 January 1854 and since no obituary has appeared as yet in The Times, one must assume that he is still alive and in good health despite his age of more than 150 years. Unconfirmed reports assert that he is now active as a bee-cultivator in Sussex.

There are a large number of textbooks on EBM. Many of them are of high quality but have the disadvantage of being too comprehensive to provide a good initial foundation for the subject. They overshoot the mark as far as most students and health care professionals are concerned. It is against this background that this handbook on EBM came about. It has been written primarily for medical and other health care students, but also for persons already working in health care.

This handbook is organized in such a way that the reader is led step by step through a process starting with a patient's medical history and leading, via information searches and critical appraisal, to a treatment recommendation. The handbook lays no claim to being all-embracing but rather is aimed at giving an introduction to EBM. A list of publications for further study is presented at the end of the manual. This would suggest that the famous quote, "Elementary, my Dear Watson", might apply to this handbook on the fundamentals of EBM, but that would be to do Holmes an injustice. In fact, this quote does not appear anywhere in the Sherlock Holmes stories; it is only a myth. But EBM is not a myth: it is a valuable tool for achieving an updated health care service based on scientific data.

The EBM process consists of four steps: "FIRE".

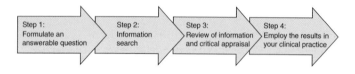

Step 1:
Formulate an answerable question

Step 2:
Information search

Step 3:
Review of information and critical appraisal

Step 4:
Employ the results in your clinical practice

Remember FIRE. The different steps in the process will be illustrated in the following sections.

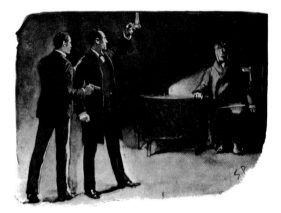

When a doctor does wrong he is the first of criminals.
He has nerve and he has knowledge.
Sherlock Holmes in *The Adventure of the Speckled Band.*

STEP 1
Formulate an
Answerable Question

The first step in the EBM process is to *F*ormulate a focused question (*F*IRE). A well-formulated question is a prerequisite for getting a useful answer. The question must be specific and concrete in order to be searchable in databases and capable of being answered after a critical appraisal of the available information. The formulation of an answerable question is neither perfectly obvious nor easy; it is a matter of finding, among tens of thousands of articles, information that best answers a clinical question pertaining to a specific patient, action or diagnostic test.

When formulating clinical questions the "PICO" approach can be used, defining the patient, intervention, comparator, and outcome [1].

P = Patient, population or problem

Which type of patient is the focus of interest, i.e. what is the patient diagnosis, population or problem?

The subject in most EBM issues is a patient with a particular diagnosis. Try to be as exact as possible in your characterization: diagnosis, stage of the illness if known, age, gender, etc. The subject may, however, also be a diagnostic test or clinical measure.

I = Intervention

What is the intervention (often the new alternative) with which you wish to compare the standard treatment, i.e. what experiment group is it?

Is the intervention a new drug, surgery, radiotherapy, etc.? Is the intervention a new diagnostic test, a new surgical method, acupuncture, etc.?

C = Comparator

What do you want to compare the intervention with? What is the control arm?

Your control is probably the treatment, test or action that is standard or most common today. Is the current standard a drug, surgical treatment, physiotherapy, etc.? Or perhaps the alternative hitherto has been not to give any treatment at all? Then a placebo may be the alternative with which the new treatment can be compared.

O = Outcome

What outcome(s) are you interested in? Does your question apply to such outcomes as survival, symptom reduction, quality of life, reduced sick-listed time, side-effects, relapses, etc.? Are health-economic effects involved? Is a new diagnostic test cheaper or more reliable?

Remember **PICO**!

Your well-thought-out question will now be used in the standard table below. It is the starting point for the formulation of your question (Step 1) and for your information search (Step 2):

		P **Patient diagnosis/ Problem**	I **Intervention**	C **Control, standard**	O **Outcome**
Step 1 F Formulate a question	Your clinical data, queries				
Step 2 I Information search	Your own search words/ textwords				
	MeSH terms				
Step 3 R Review of information and critical appraisal					
Step 4 E Employ the results					

EXAMPLE

Let's take an example to illustrate how the standard table can be used.

In *The Hound of the Baskervilles*, the body of Sir Charles Baskerville was found on the Devonshire Moor with features convulsed with some strong emotion and an almost incredible facial distortion. It was assumed that Sir Charles had tried to escape from someone or something – perhaps a hound – and succumbed to a cardiac event. Dr Mortimer, the deceased's friend and medical attendant, described Sir Charles as a retiring man who had the habit of smoking cigars and that there was a history of impaired health that pointed to some affection of the heart. From this information we may deduce that Sir Charles was affected by angina pectoris and probably had experienced myocardial infarction prior to his fatal cardiac event.

On a popular health care website (Medical Link with over 70,000 visitors per month) there is information stating that vitamin E can reduce the risk of dying of myocardial infarction by 77% – an impressive figure! Had Dr Mortimer been aware of this information he might have considered treating Sir Charles with vitamin E; or would he not? Let us use the EBM process to see what the scientific literature says about this.

In Step 2 (p. 19ff.), we shall use these clinical data for an information search.

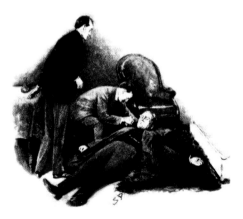

There is nothing more deceptive than an obvious fact.
Sherlock Holmes in *The Boscombe Valley Mystery.*

Fill in clinical data in the standard table:

		P **Patient** **diagnosis/** **Problem**	**I** **Intervention**	**C** **Control,** **standard**	**O** **Outcome**
Step 1 **F** Formulate a question	Your clinical data, queries	*65+-year-old* *male, angina* *pectoris,* *myocardial* *infarction*	*Vitamins,* *vitamin E*	*No vitamins*	*New* *infarction,* *death*
Step 2 **I** Information search	Your own search words/ textwords				
	MeSH terms				
Step 3 **R** Review of information and critical appraisal					
Step 4 **E** Employ the results					

Information resources

After you have formulated a question or defined a problem, the next step is to try to find relevant information by means of electronic data searches. However, the quantity of information available on the Web can be overwhelming and information from some websites may be biased, out-of-date or of poor quality. The key to efficient searching is to know where reliable and relevant information can be found most often.

In principle, there are four different sources of information:
- *Systematic reviews/meta-analyses*: These secondary sources of information consist of compilations of original articles that have been vetted by

independent researchers and clinicians. The most important vetting organization is the Cochrane Collaboration.
- *Clinical Practice Guidelines*: These reviews deal with large disease groups and treatment strategies.
- *Critically Appraised Topics (CATs)*: A CAT is a short summary of evidence on a specific clinical question.
- *Original articles containing primary data*: What is of interest here is mainly original articles based on randomized-controlled trials (RCTs).

Choosing the appropriate database

The type of information source and search strategy to choose depends on the subject area (medicine, dentistry, occupational therapy, etc.) and the type of question being asked (drug effect, diagnostic problem, screening issue, etc.). Questions pertaining to treatment alternatives or therapeutic effects involving common illnesses can often be found in the systematic reviews/meta-analyses. General recommendations pertaining to more common illnesses can be found in the Clinical Practice Guidelines and answers to specific clinical issues may sometimes be found among CATs. More special issues and new research findings are chiefly dealt with in original articles.

You should always begin your search with the secondary information sources since independent examiners have already vetted the basic scientific material. Because of the size and complexity of MEDLINE, searching this database as a first option is a less attractive alternative unless your question is a very specific and research-oriented one.

The following order of search steps is likely to be successful for most EBM purposes:
1 Try Cochrane Library (p. 6f.).
2 Make a meta-engine search (p. 9f.).
3 Explore secondary information databases including Clinical Queries (p. 7f.) and CATs (p. 14).
4 Go to Clinical Practice Guideline databases (p. 11f.).
5 Use MEDLINE (PubMed) and other primary information sources (p. 14f.).

The various databases are presented in the following sections.

Systematic reviews/meta-analyses

A systematic review summarizes a concrete clinical question, in which an attempt has been made to avoid any systematic error (*bias*), and a meta-analysis is a review using a quantitative methodology to summarize the results of different studies. The feature that secondary information sources have in common is that the information is based on an analysis of a number of individual scientific studies (primary information sources) which have been appraised scientifically and supplemented with a summarizing assessment of the results of the various studies. There are quite a number of thorough and reliable systematic information sources compiled and updated by professional or public authorities, e.g. the Cochrane Collaboration and Health Technology Assessment (HTA) agencies. Some are free of charge on the Web (WWW), some have been purchased for free use by teaching staff and students at particular universities, while others require a subscription (£).

The Cochrane Library (£)

The Cochrane Library is the most important secondary source of information and thus it is best to start a search there. The Cochrane Collaboration is an international professional organization that compiles systematic reviews in important fields of medicine. Strict criteria are used in its evaluations and its published reports are characterized by high quality and reliability. A subscription is required for full access but most health science libraries have subscriptions and some countries have open access agreements to make it freely available in their country.

The Cochrane Library is a collection of databases that contain high quality, independent evidence to inform healthcare decision making. In addition to Cochrane Reviews, which is the most important database, The Cochrane Library provides other sources of reliable information, i.e. technology assessments, economical evaluations and individual clinical trials, all in one same environment. **www.thecochranelibrary.com**

- *Cochrane Reviews* contain about 4000 complete systematic reviews of the highest quality. The reviews summarize conclusions about effectiveness and provide a unique collection of known evidence on a given topic. The full reviews are complete with results and discussion, meta-analysis and odds-ratio diagrams. The protocols are outlines of reviews in preparation including the background, rationale and methods.
- *Other Reviews* includes about 6000 structured abstracts of systematic reviews from around the world which have been evaluated by reviewers at the Centre for Reviews and Dissemination (CRD) in the UK. Only reviews that meet minimum quality criteria are included. These reviews cover topics that have yet to be addressed in Cochrane Reviews.
- *Clinical Trials* includes details of about 450,000 RCTs retrieved by reviewers in the Cochrane Collaboration. Records include the title of the article,

bibliographic details and, in many cases, a summary of the article. They do not contain the full text of the article.
- *Technology Assessments* contains details about 4000 ongoing projects and completed publications. Records do not include the full text of the report but some have structured abstracts or indications where further details can be obtained.

Clinical Queries in PubMed

The second-best source of systematic reviews after Cochrane is MEDLINE/PubMed. PubMed will be described in more detail further on pp. 20–31, but here we shall focus on PubMed's ability to retrieve systematic reviews via the Clinical Queries function. PubMed is accessible free of charge via the home pages of most university libraries or directly via **www.pubmed.gov**. In the blue side bar to the left on the home page, you will see the heading *Clinical Queries.* Click on it and then click in the circle in front of Systematic Reviews. Then fill in your search word in the white query box.

Clinical Queries uses filters that combine your search with a few select MeSH headings (Medical Subject Headings) (see pp. 20–21) to filter searches for: *Therapy, Diagnosis, Etiology* or *Prognosis.* The search filters included in Clinical Queries are useful for EBM purposes since they filter out unwanted articles. If you want to do a wide search, you should select *Sensitivity* (at the risk of getting many irrelevant hits). If you want to do a narrower search, you should click on *Specificity* (at the risk of missing relevant articles).

The Clinical Queries function has been created to facilitate the retrieval of systematic reviews, meta-analyses, quality-assessed articles, articles in the area of EBM, Clinical Practice Guidelines, consensus reports, etc. The function has a sensitivity of 93–97% for identifying high-quality systematic reviews published in Cochrane and the ACP Journal Club [3]. You should realize, however, that only about 50% of the references retrieved meet current requirements for systematic reviews. The remaining references are made up of reviews of more doubtful quality. A search in PubMed limited to "review articles" (within the *Limits* function; see p. 28) is a less attractive alternative because the high-quality systematic reviews will constitute less than 10% of the references obtained here [3].

Bandolier

Bandolier contains concise and readily accessible systematic reviews of therapy studies, diagnostic tests, epidemiological and health-economy studies. Bandolier comprises some 3000 systematic reviews. **www.jr2.ox.ac.uk/bandolier**

CRD

CRD comprises about 100 systematic reviews of common medical problems and disorders. **www.york.ac.uk/inst/crd**

Secondary information sources (systematic reviews)

Database	Access via	Authorization
Cochrane Library	**www.thecochranelibrary.com**	Subscription; free in some countries
Clinical Queries	**www.pubmed.gov**	Free
Bandolier	**www.jr2.ox.ac.uk/bandolier**	Free
CRD databases	**www.york.ac.uk/inst/crd**	Free

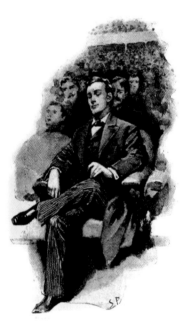

You see, but you do not observe.
Holmes to Watson in *A Scandal in Bohemia.*

Meta-search engines

Several useful meta-search engines are available. They search multiple databases and provide information from bibliographic databases from different health science fields, data from universities and from government and regulatory agencies, as well as from commercial bodies. They also search different categories of information including original/primary studies, systematic reviews and Clinical Practice Guidelines. The meta-search engines TRIP (Turning Research into Practice Database) and SUMSearch are very useful and are highly recommended. The general meta-search engine Google and the science-focused search tool Scirus can also provide useful medical information but critical appraisal of the provided information is essential.

TRIP (£)

TRIP is a meta-search engine that searches a large number of highly reliable databases. It contains clinical guidance sites, CATs databases, systematic review collections and other EBM products including E-textbooks and medical images. Non-subscribers are limited to three free searches. **www.tripdatabase.com**

SUMSearch

SUMSearch combines different search strategies and uses several different search engines. It provides a good overview of review articles, clinical guidelines, systematic reviews and original articles. One very useful function of SUMSearch is that you can check your search word against the MeSH terms on which searches with SUMSearch are based ("Check my strategy"). **http://sumsearch.uthscsa.edu**

Scirus

This is a search engine that focuses on web pages with a scientific content and locates scientific, scholarly, technical and medical data included in journals and university and government sites and filters out non-scientific sites. A useful function is the provision of keywords identified by your primary search that enable you to refine your search. **www.scirus.com**

Google

This large general meta-search engine is surprisingly good for EBM purposes and contains many links to EBM resources, EBM search tools, electronic calculators and sometimes also high-quality studies. A careful quality appraisal is required, however. **www.google.com**

A useful list of various EBM resources as well as an EBM search tool may be found at **http://directory.google.com** go to Health → Medicine → Evidence Based Medicine.

Meta-search engines

Database	Access via	Authorization
TRIP Database	**www.tripdatabase.com**	Subscription
SUMSearch	**http://sumsearch.uthscsa.edu**	Free
Scirus	**www.scirus.com**	Free
Google	**www.google.com**	Free

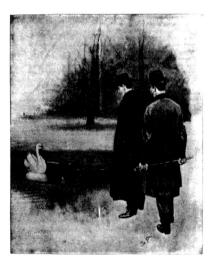

I never guess. It is a shocking habit, destructive to the logical faculty. What seems strange to you is only so because you do not follow my train of thought or observe the small facts upon which large inferences may depend.
Holmes to Watson in *The Science of Deduction.*

Clinical Practice Guidelines

Clinical Practice Guidelines often give a good overview in important areas of medicine, but their quality varies and, in many instances, you will not get an answer to more specific queries. The use of Clinical Practice Guidelines therefore requires you to evaluate the contents with regard to reliability and relevance and to judge the way in which the information can be applied to your own clinical reality. There are a number of excellent Clinical Practice Guidelines. Most of them require a subscription (£), but some are freely accessible on the Web.

Clinical Evidence (£)

Clinical Evidence is issued by the British Medical Journal (BMJ) and is a brief summary of the current state of knowledge regarding the prevention and treatment of common clinical conditions. It is published in book form every 6 months and is available in its entirety on the Web. Clinical Evidence proceeds from important clinical queries and summarizes the available information. In this respect, Clinical Evidence differs from, e.g. Cochrane and therefore constitutes a good complement. **www.clinicalevidence.com**

EBM Guidelines (£)

EBM Guidelines comprise over 1000 Clinical Practice Guidelines covering a wide range of diseases, primarily in the field of general medicine. It also contains a large collection of pictures of skin diseases. The scientific strength of the treatment recommendations is indicated (A: strong research-based evidence; B: moderate; C: limited; D: no research-based evidence). **www.ebm-guidelines.com**

FIRSTConsult (£)

This Clinical Practice Guideline is produced by Elsevier and is an evidence-graded resource providing information about evaluation, therapy, diagnosis, outcomes and prevention. It is very large and offers coverage of hundreds of different conditions and of over 800 medical topics as well as information on drugs, therapies and complaints. **www.firstconsult.com**

NeLH

NeLH (National Electronic Library for Health) is a gateway to a large number of electronic resources and it provides many useful links (to Clinical

Evidence, Cochrane Library, Bandolier, NICE (The National Institute for Health and Clinical Excellence), PRODIGY, among others). The Guidelines Finder holds details of over 1500 UK national guidelines.
www.nelh.nhs.uk

NICE

NICE is a part of the NHS (National Health Service) and provides guidance for clinical practice, health technology, interventional procedures and public health. More than 400 appraisals are available on the website.
www.nice.org.uk

PRODIGY

PRODIGY is an NHS database providing guidance on common conditions and symptoms often seen in primary care. The summary of evidence and best clinical practice is presented for each condition together with recommendations for management. The guidance is structured to support decision-making in the consultation and is written in a succinct style.
www.prodigy.nhs.uk

NGC

NGC (National Guideline Clearinghouse) is a large, well-made database comprising evidence-based Clinical Practice Guidelines provided by the US Department of Health. It contains several thousand clinical guidelines pertaining to illnesses and diseases, as well as treatments and interventions.
www.guidelines.gov

PIER (£)

PIER (Physician's Information and Education Resource) is an evidence-based guide produced by the American College of Physicians. It covers individual diseases, legal medicine, ethics, complementary/alternative medicine, common procedures, screening and prevention. PIER rates its recommendations based on the underlying evidence and each citation by the evidence level. The database contains specific recommendations, abstracts and, in some cases, full-text versions of related clinical material.
http://pier.acponline.org

Clinical Practice Guidelines

Database	Access via	Authorization
Clinical Evidence	**www.clinicalevidence.com**	Subscription
EBM Guidelines	**www.ebm-guidelines.com**	Subscription
FIRSTConsult	**www.firstconsult.com**	Subscription
NeLH	**www.nelh.nhs.uk**	Free
NICE	**www.nice.org.uk**	Free
PRODIGY	**www.prodigy.nhs.uk**	Free
NGC	**www.guidelines.gov**	Free
PIER	**http://pier.acponline.org**	Subscription
UptoDate	**www.uptodate.com**	Subscription

1
2
3
4

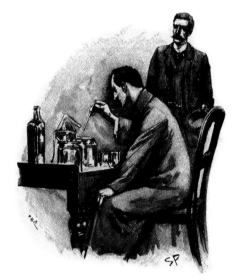

It is a capital mistake to theorize before one has data. Insensibly one begins to twist facts to suit theories, instead of theories to suit facts.
Sherlock Holmes in *A Scandal in Bohemia.*

Critically Appraised topics (CATs)

A CAT is a short summary of evidence regarding a clinical question. It is like a shorter and less rigorous version of a systematic review, summarizing the best evidence on a topic. At some centres, CATs are used as a university assignment to assess students' skills and knowledge. The Evidence-Based Medicine Journal and ACP Journal Club publish material based on article reviews (see p. 14ff.) and are similar to the topic reviews of CATs.

There are a large number of CAT sites available on the Web:
- BestBETS (emergency medicine topics): **www.bestbets.org**
- CAT Crawler (a CAT search engine): **www.bii-sg.org**; search: CAT Crawler
- Centre for EBM, Oxford (general topics): **www.cebm.net**
- Evidence-Based on-call: **www.eboncall.org**
- Neurology CATs: **www.uwo.ca**; search: Neurology CATs
- Evidence-based pediatrics Website: **www.med.umich.edu/pediatrics/ebm**
- Family practice CATs: **www.cfpc.ca/english/cfpc/clfm/critical**
- Scottish Intensive Care Society: **www.sicsebm.org.uk**
- Occupational therapy: **www.otcats.com**

Primary information sources

PubMed

PubMed is one of several other interfaces (e.g. OVID) connected to the largest biomedical database: MEDLINE. Knowledge of PubMed and its search technique can be used in searches in other medical databases. PubMed can be accessed free of charge via the National Library of Medicine (NLM) and contains about 16 million references to articles in 4800 biomedical journals. Most of the references are accompanied by abstracts and, in some cases, the whole article is available. Owing to its size and complex contents, PubMed demands knowledge of its structure and appropriate search strategies. **www.pubmed.gov**

How a search in PubMed is carried out is described on pp. 20–33. PubMed contains the important MeSH function (described in more detail on pp. 20–31).

EMBASE (£)

This database covers 6500 journals, including 2000 not covered by MEDLINE. It covers pharmacology and biomedicine in general, notably drug literature, physical and rehabilitation medicine and occupational and physical therapy. EMBASE is a good supplement to MEDLINE as these two databases have different selection criteria and indexing policies. **www.embase.com**

Primary information sources

Database	Access via	Authorization	Subject matter
MEDLINE			
PubMed:	**www.pubmed.gov**	Free	Medicine, bioscience,
OVID:	**http://gateway.ovid.com**	Subscription	education, health care
EMBASE	**www.embase.com**	Subscription	Medicine, pharmacology, nursing care
CINAHL	**www.cinahl.com**	Subscription	Physiotherapy, occupational therapy, nutrition
AMED	**www.bl.uk; search: AMED**	Subscription	Alternative medicine, physical therapy, occupational therapy, rehabilitation, palliative care
National Cancer Institute	**www.cancer.gov**	Free	Cancer
Psycinfo	**www.apa.org/psycinfo**	Subscription	Psychiatry, psychology

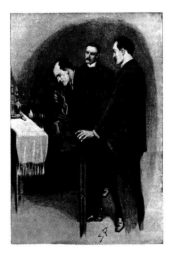

You know by method. It is founded upon the observance of trifles.
Sherlock Holmes in *The Boscombe Valley Mystery.*

Library resources

University libraries

Important EBM resources are available to students and teachers at their respective universities. The selection comprises a large number of databases and electronically available full-text journals.

MEDLINE (PubMed or Ovid), the Cochrane Library and thousands of electronic journals are standard at all large university libraries as well as the databases EMBASE, CINAHL, AMED, Psycinfo and more.

University libraries are the rich sources of various EBM products including databases, journals and EBM tutorials. The list below contains a selected sample of universities that have been particularly active in promoting EBM (use the search function at each site for EBM information):

- University of Toronto: **www.utoronto.ca**
- University of Oxford: **www.ox.ac.uk**
- University of York: **www.york.ac.uk**
- University of Sheffield: **www.shef.ac.uk**
- Duke University: **www.duke.edu**
- University of Alberta: **www.ualberta.ca**
- University of Sidney: **www.usyd.edu.au**

Other EBM portals

INAHTA

The INAHTA (International Network of Agencies for Health Technology Assessment) site includes links to over 40 national HTA agencies worldwide. Many high-quality sites can be found here. **www.inahta.org**

NLM

NLM provides a wide selection of databases and articles with abstracts or in full text, as well as clinical guidelines and health care information for the general public. The most important ones are MEDLINE/PubMed, NLM Gateway, MEDLINEplus, HSTAT and National Cancer Institute website. **www.nlm.nih.gov**

EBM online (£)

This is the website for the Evidence-Based Medicine Journal. Clinical experts review and comment on original and review articles of particular importance to clinical care. It covers important advances in internal medicine, general and family practice, surgery, psychiatry, paediatrics, gynaecology and obstetrics. **http://ebm.bmjjournals.com**

ACP Journal Club (£)

This database is generated using procedures identical to those used for the Evidence-Based Medicine Journal. The contents are selected from over 100 journals using explicit criteria for scientific merit followed by assessments of relevance to medical practice. **www.acpjc.org**

Netting the evidence

Comprehensive overview of EBM resources on the Internet as well as useful learning resources. Produced by ScHARR, University of Sheffield. **www.shef.ac.uk/scharr/ir/netting**

AHRQ

The AHRQ (Agency for Healthcare Research and Quality) in the US produces evidence-based practice programmes for many different conditions. **www.ahcpr.gov/clinic/epcindex.htm**

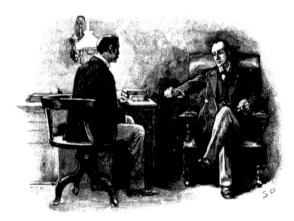

The temptation to form premature theories upon insufficient data is the bane of our profession.
Sherlock Holmes in *The Tragedy of Birlstone.*

STEP 2
Information Search

The second step in EBM is searching for *I*nformation (F*I*RE) on the Web. It is important to realize that there are many different search pathways and not one "absolutely right" search outcome. So try different search methods to find articles of interest. The overarching strategy in database searches is first to do as wide a search as possible to increase the probability of the articles you are interested in being included (secure a high level of sensitivity) and then apply restrictions to eliminate articles that you are not interested in (increase the specificity). The goal is to retrieve all relevant articles (100% sensitivity) but no irrelevant ones (100% specificity) – a goal which is of course impossible to fully achieve. In this section you will see an example of how you can reduce an initial "hit" comprising more than one million references to just 27.

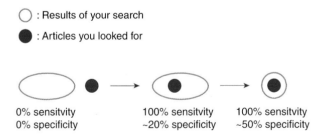

The main steps of the search procedure in PubMed and other databases are as follows:

1 Do a wide search (secure a high level of sensitivity in your search).
2 Restrict your search results and reduce the number of irrelevant hits (increase the specificity).
3 Use a good hit to find other relevant articles.

Make a wide search with high sensitivity

In order to make a wide search, it is necessary to try different strategies, check the outcome and follow-up items that seem to work. Again, there is no "absolutely right" outcome and you have to proceed by trial and error. There are two main search strategies and you should make use of both of them:

- Free textword searches in which you use your own search terms.
- Searches with MeSH terms, which constitute a specific indexing and classification system used by medical libraries and in databases.

Free textword searches

Searches using free textwords (keywords or phrases) can be made in most databases, but we will illustrate this with PubMed. Visit PubMed's home page **www.pubmed.gov** and enter one or more words in the query box at the top of the page. You can use small letters throughout. Click on GO, whereupon PubMed will combine your words automatically (AND is inserted automatically between the words). The number of hits is shown and you will be presented with a number of references. Most of the references in PubMed include an abstract of the article, which you can call up by clicking on the underlined names of the authors. Some articles are presented in their entirety and these can be called up by clicking on the name of the publisher immediately above the heading of the article. For most textwords PubMed will automatically link to a MeSH term (check by clicking on the *Details* function to confirm). PubMed (and also TRIP and Scirus databases) will sometimes suggest alternative search words.

Searching by textwords can be effective as long as you include all the various synonyms for your search (see p. 22).

Searching with MeSH

MeSH terms constitute a specific indexing and classification system consisting of controlled subject headings used to describe the contents of each article entered in MEDLINE. MeSH stands for *Medical Subject Headings* and is a kind of bibliographical dictionary or thesaurus used to enable computers to understand what you are looking for. There are about 22,000 MeSH terms in the system and you should use them to avoid missing relevant articles.

MeSH terms are classified in different subject groups and are arranged hierarchically, e.g.:

All MeSH Categories
    Diseases Category
        Cardiovascular Diseases
            Vascular Diseases
                Ischemia
                    Myocardial Ischemia
                        Myocardial Infarction
                            Myocardial Stunning
                                Shock, Cardiogenic

Thus *cardiovascular diseases* range higher up in the hierarchy than *myocardial infarction* so that a search on this word will usually also include *myocardial infarction*. PubMed automatically includes all MeSH terms that range below the MeSH term you have chosen (i.e. an *Explode* function is also included). Therefore, always check that your search word is a MeSH term, where it ranges in the hierarchy and if there is a MeSH term higher up in the hierarchy that may be even more useful. Go to PubMed's home page **www.pubmed.gov** and click on *MeSH Database* listed in the side bar. Enter a textword. If your textword is not a MeSH term, suggestions for such will be provided.

Combining terms and sets

After creating sets of citations that are pertinent to your topic you may want to combine two or more of these sets. If you want to use search words with similar meanings, you should combine them by typing, for instance, *smoking* OR *tobacco*. You will then be presented with articles that are indexed with either *smoking* or *tobacco*. This search strategy is called Boolean search (after its creator George Boole). The terms OR, AND and NOT have the following meanings:

Boolean operators				Meaning
OR:	Smoking		Tobacco	Retrieves articles with either word
AND:	Breast neoplasms		Risk factors	Retrieves articles with *both* words
NOT:	Breast neoplasms		Male cancer	Retrieves articles with some exclusion

Principal database search strategy

Under the search area (query box) in the upper portion of PubMed's starting page you will find the Features Bar with the following headings: *Limits, Preview/Index, History, Clipboard, Details*. The *Limits* function is described in more detail on p. 28, but here we shall take a closer look at the *Details* and *History* functions.

Details

This function shows how your search has been translated by PubMed's automatic term mapping of the *MeSH terms, Subheadings* and *Text Words* that have been used and how your search terms have been combined with AND, OR and NOT, respectively. When searching in PubMed, an automatic search is made for similar subject terms. After searching on heart attack, the *Details*

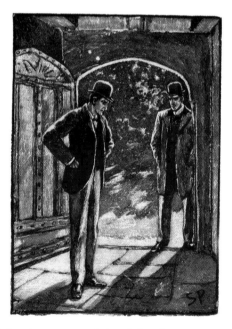

When you follow two separate chains of thought, Watson, you will find some intersection which should approximate to the truth.
Sherlock Holmes in *The Disappearance of Lady Frances Carfax.*

function will show *myocardial infarction [MeSH term]* OR *heart attack [Text Word]*. This means that the search on *heart attack* results in the automatic inclusion of the MeSH term *myocardial infarction*. Use *Details* any time you want to check how PubMed understood the search terms you entered.

History

PubMed will hold all your search strategies and results in *History*. It displays the search number, your search query and the number of citations in your results. To view the results from a search, click on the number of results.

The *History* function is very useful for combining several search terms. The general method for database searching is based on PICO (pp. 1–2) as follows:

$$P \ \text{AND} \ I \ \text{AND} \ C \ \text{AND} \ O$$

However, since each of the *P, I, C, O* parts may have several synonyms (typically two or three), each of the four parts need to be explored separately to obtain the maximum search outcome. Your search strategy should therefore be (assuming one synonym for each *P, I, C, O* part):

$$(P_1 \ \text{OR} \ P_2) \ \text{AND} \ (I_1 \ \text{OR} \ I_2) \ \text{AND} \ (C_1 \ \text{OR} \ C_2) \ \text{AND} \ (O_1 \ \text{OR} \ O_2)$$

PubMed's *History* function is very useful for refining search strategies by adding one or more terms, one at a time. Click on *History* and do your search as follows:

Write	Command 1	PubMed Table will show: "Most recent Queries"	Command 2
Your P_1-word	PREVIEW	#1	CLEAR
Your P_2-word	PREVIEW	#2	CLEAR
All *P*s: #1 AND #2	PREVIEW	#3	CLEAR
Repeat procedure for all synonyms also for your I, C and O, yielding:			
All *I*s: #4 AND #5	PREVIEW	#6	CLEAR
All *C*s: # 7 AND #8	PREVIEW	#9	CLEAR
All *O*s: #10 AND #11	PREVIEW	#12	CLEAR

Finally, write: #3 AND #6 AND #9 AND #12, click on PREVIEW and the combined result of your search will be shown (=#13).

It is usually not necessary to include a search on C (Control) if, for instance, *RCT* is included in the search; as then, by definition, there must be a control group anyhow. Check with the *Details* function to see how your search was interpreted. Click on the hits result and the references you have found with your search will be shown. If your search has yielded 0 (nil) hits, it is probable that you have either made some mistake (e.g. misspelled), taken the process too far or, alternatively, there are no articles available on your query (which is highly unlikely). If you have obtained too many hits (more than 300–400) you may need to improve the specificity of your search (see p. 27).

EXAMPLE

Now we will do a broad search by choosing free textwords that are relevant to your subject. Let us return to the example (on p. 3) where Dr Mortimer wondered about the effect of vitamin E on the risk of dying of myocardial infarction. (As always, you will have first done a search in the Cochrane Library and found that no complete report is available, but a protocol was being developed [4].) You should now fill in the standard table with your own search terms. Use medical textwords of your own which you consider to be relevant to your question. Try to think of different words with similar meanings for each of your P, I ,C, O words, (e.g. cardiac arrest, cardiac asystole, cardiac standstill, coronary attack, heart arrest, myocardial necrosis).

Fill in clinical data in the standard table:

		P **Patient diagnosis/ problem**	**I** **Intervention**	**C** **Control, standard**	**O** **Outcome**
Step 1 **F** Formulate a question	Your clinical data, queries	*65+ -year-old male, angina pectoris, myocardial infarction*	*Vitamins, vitamin E*	*No vitamins*	*New infarction, death*
Step 2 **I** Information search	Your own search words/ textwords MeSH terms	*Angina pectoris, myocardial infarction, heart attack, cardiac arrest, cardiac standstill, etc.*	*Vitamins, vitamin E, antioxidants, free radicals, oxidative stress, scavengers*	*Control, placebo*	*Death, mortality*
Step 3 **R** Review of information and critical appraisal					
Step 4 **E** Employ the results					

The next step is to find appropriate MeSH terms (pp. 20–21).
Fill in the MeSH terms in the standard table:

		P **Patient diagnosis/ Problem**	I **Intervention**	C **Control, standard**	O **Outcome**
Step 1 F Formulate a question	Your clinical data, queries	*65+ -year-old male, angina pectoris, myocardial infarction*	*Vitamins, vitamin E*	*No vitamins*	*New infarction, death*
Step 2 I Information search	Your own search words/ textwords	*Angina pectoris, myocardial infarction, heart attack, cardiac arrest, cardiac standstill, etc.*	*Vitamins, vitamin E, antioxidants, free radicals, oxidative stress, scavengers*	*Control, placebo*	*Death, mortality*
	MeSH terms	*Myocardial infarction, angina pectoris, arteriosclerosis*	*Vitamins, vitamin E, antioxidants, free radicals*	*Control, placebo*	*Death, mortality*
Step 3 R Review of information and critical appraisal					
Step 4 E Employ the results					

Determine what MeSH terms are higher up in the hierarchy by opening PubMed's home page via **www.pubmed.gov**. Click on *MeSH Database* in the blue side bar to the left on the starting page. Check the position of your particular MeSH terms in the hierarchy by entering them in the white box at the top. Here you can also get definitions of the terms and find alternative terms or similar concepts. For example, there is a reference to antioxidants for vitamin E. The following information will be presented.

MeSH term	MeSH term higher up in the hierarchy or referenced MeSH terms
Myocardial infarction	Cardiovascular diseases
Angina pectoris	Cardiovascular diseases
Arteriosclerosis	Cardiovascular diseases
Vitamin E	Antioxidants
Free radicals	Antioxidants
Oxidative stress	Antioxidants
Scavengers	Antioxidants
Death	Death
Mortality	Mortality

A search for the combination *cardiovascular disease* AND *antioxidants* AND (*death* OR *mortality*) results in over 1000 hits. Articles relevant to your query will probably be among them (good sensitivity), but the problem is that they will be concealed among many articles that you are not interested in (poor specificity).

Limit your search results/increase your specificity

Hopefully, you will now have retrieved articles that can answer your query (i.e. you have achieved good sensitivity). The next step will be to increase your search specificity by restricting your search by trying to exclude the articles you have retrieved but in which you are not interested. The terms AND or NOT increase the specificity of your search (p. 21).

Limits

Use PubMed's *Limits* function positioned in the Feature bar below the white query box. This function reduces the number of hits by allowing you to restrict your search. You can limit your search to a specific age group or gender, a specific language or to specific types of articles such as RCTs. The most useful restrictions in the *Limits* function are the following:

Limitation	Example
Publication types	Clinical trial
	Meta-analysis
	Practice Guideline
	Randomized controlled trial
	Review
Language	English
Human or animal	Human
Entrez date	5 years

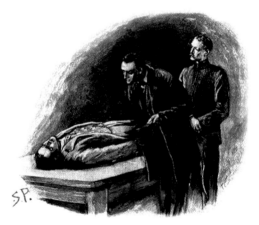

It is an old maxim of mine that when you have excluded the impossible, whatever remains, however improbable, must be the truth.
Holmes in *The Adventure of the Beryl Coronet.*

SLIM

A recent development in PubMed is the alternative Web interface SLIM (Slider Interface for MEDLINE/PubMed searches). SLIM uses five different interactive slider bars to control various search parameters such as limits, filters and MeSH terminologies. SLIM is intended to improve user control and the capability to instantly refine and refocus search strategies [5]. **http://pmi.nlm.nih.gov/slide**

Useful suffixes in PubMed (Note: You must use square brackets):

Suffix	Meaning	Example
[au]	Author	Smith [au]
[ta]	Journal title abbreviation	Lancet [ta]
[mh]	MeSH term	breast neoplasms [mh]
[pt]	Publication type	review [pt]
[tw]	Textword (word in title of article or abstract)	breast cancer [tw]
[ti]	Title (word in title of article)	risk factor [ti]
[sb]	MeSH Subheadings (describes a particular aspect of a subject)	therapeutic use [sb]
*	Truncation (searches for main stem of word)	staph*
" "	Quotation marks (search for exact search term)	"health planning"
( )	Connects words	hyperparathyroidism NOT (renal OR secondary)

Useful MeSH terms when searching for therapy studies, diagnostic tests, systematic reviews / meta-analyses and Clinical Practice Guidelines, respectively:

	Useful MeSH terms
Therapy studies	Randomized controlled trial [pt]
	Controlled clinical trial [pt]
	Clinical trial [pt]
	Meta-analysis [pt]
	Random [tw]
	Random* [ta]
	Placebo
	Prognosis
	Therapeutic use [sb]
	Morbidity
	Mortality
Diagnostic tests	Sensitivity [tw]
	Specificity [tw]
	Predictive value [tw]
	Likelihood functions
	Diagnosis, differential
Systematic reviews/meta-analysis	Review [pt]
	Meta-analysis [pt]
	Odds ratio – prognosis
	Systematic [sb]
	Morbidity
	Mortality
Clinical Practice Guidelines	Guidelines [tw]
	Guideline* [tw]
	Practice guideline
	Guide [tw]
	Recommend* [tw]

EXAMPLE

Now if we return to the example (on p. 3 and p. 25ff.) and Dr Mortimer's query about the effect of antioxidants on cardiovascular disease, the result of a PubMed search (displayed in the *History* function) will be as follows:

Search term	Number of hits
Cardiovascular diseases (#1)	>1 million
Antioxidants (#2)	>100,000
Death OR mortality (#3)	>600,000
#1 AND #2 AND #3	>1000

It seems that a search covering cardiovascular diseases, antioxidants, death and mortality has the prerequisites for yielding many hits with high sensitivity. But the specificity needs to be increased. Using study-type specific MeSH terms can do this.

Randomized controlled trial (#4)	>200,000
Meta-analysis (#5)	>14,000

You can then combine the above search terms by writing #1 AND #2, etc. in the search box:

Combined search words	Number of hits
#1 AND #2	>9000
#1 AND #2 AND #3	>1000
#1 AND #2 AND #3 AND #4	239
#1 AND #2 AND #3 AND #5	27

Thus, by combining the MeSH terms *cardiovascular diseases* AND *antioxidants* AND (*death* OR *mortality*) AND *meta-analysis* as search words, you have come down from over 1 million hits to 27 articles.

On examining these 27 hits, we find the article by Vivekananthan et al., Use of antioxidant vitamins for the prevention of cardiovascular disease: meta-analysis of randomized trials [6]. This study summarizes 12 large trials in which over 130,000 patients were studied. The conclusion drawn from the study is that vitamin E has no positive effect on cardiovascular mortality and that beta-carotene actually increases the mortality. Thus, this meta-analysis arrived at an entirely different conclusion than that presented by the commercial Website ("Vitamin E can reduce the risk of dying of myocardial infarction by 77%").

(You should also take a look at the articles retrieved ($n = 239$) with the combination #1 AND #2 AND #3 AND #4. There may be articles here that are of interest.)

Use a good hit for further searches

The next step in the search procedure is to look through the articles you have retrieved, select a relevant one and use it to find other articles of interest. Let's continue with PubMed.

Related Articles

Once you have found an article that is relevant, click on the Related Articles function to the right of the article. The function yields hits on articles that are indexed similarly to the article you have identified. In our example, we get more than 100 such Related Articles proceeding from the article by Vivekananthan et al. [6].

It may also be a good idea to check the MeSH terms with which the retrieved article is indexed: Go to the Display function and select the Citation format and you will be presented with the MeSH [mh] terms with which the identified article was indexed. You can use these MeSH terms to find similar articles.

Once you have found an article of interest, you can check out the summary (abstract) by clicking on the underscored line showing the name of the author. Some journals offer direct access to the whole article in PubMed (e.g. BMJ) so you can read it immediately or print it out (preferably in the PDF format). The university libraries subscribe to a large number of electronic versions of journals and thereby enable you to make printouts of many of the articles you have found.

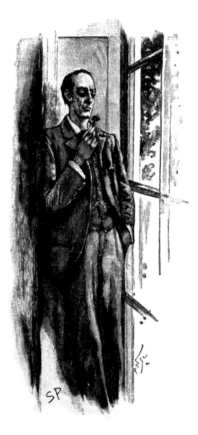

The ideal reasoner would, when he had once been shown a single fact in all its bearings, deduce from it, not only all the chains of events which led up to it, but also all the results which would follow from it.
Sherlock Holmes in *The Five Orange Pips.*

STEP 3
Review of Information and Critical Appraisal

The next step in the application of EBM is to *R*eview, and critically appraise the scientific data (FI*R*E). The ability to evaluate medical information (assess the evidence) is an important part of EBM. This process involves a systematic analysis of the validity and reliability of the information as well as of the results and relevance of the particular articles. The *validity* of a study has to do with the extent to which an analysis or investigation measures what it is intended to measure. How reliable is the study when it comes to establishing the "truth"? By the *internal validity* of a study is meant the reliability of the experimental design ("for demonstrating the truth") and by its *external validity* is meant the extent to which the results of the study can be considered applicable to the patients included in the study in question ("Can the results be applied to my patients?"). The *reliability* of a study pertains to how reproducible its results are ("If we repeat the study many times, will the results be the same?").

The meaning of the concepts validity and reliability can be illustrated by the results of a shooting practice performed by Holmes, Watson, inspectors Gregson and Lestrade that are shown on next page.

Not unexpectedly, Holmes' score was characterized by a high validity and reliability, whereas Lestrade's score had a low degree of validity as well as low reliability.

Quality assessment of information

Medical practice is guided by knowledge, experience, experimentation and value systems. These components have a variable evidence base that needs to be considered before making decisions about care in individual patients. The experience of groups of practitioners offers stronger evidence than the experience of individual caregivers, and RCTs often yield stronger evidence than observational studies.

The evaluation of various information sources to form a recommendation is a complex process that involves knowledge of the characteristics of

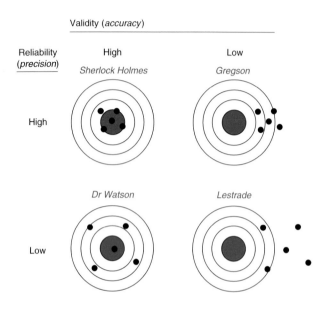

study designs, an assessment of the quality of the study and the application of the evidence to match the patient's needs and preferences [7].

In this section we shall focus on the quality assessment of the information. This process includes:

- An analysis of the study design.
- Grading the level of evidence.
- Critical appraisal.
- Grading the quality of the evidence.

The final step to reach a decision on medical intervention involves:

- An analysis of the balance between benefit and harm.
- Evaluation of the strength of a recommendation.
- Implementation.

In order to be able to use the "best research evidence" in accordance with the EBM definition, it is necessary to assess the quality of the information or investigation. There are two principal study designs that are used to establish interventional effects: experimental and observational studies.

Experimental studies are designed to minimize the risk of bias, i.e. to produce results that do not depart systematically from the truth. The best evidence for a cause and effect relationship stems from well-conducted experimental studies with a large number of patients, randomly allocated comparison groups, blinded caregivers, patients and data analysts, few patients lost to follow-up and in which methods of high quality have been used for measurements of effects and for analyzing gathered data. The study design that carries the most weight as evidence is the RCT.

Observational studies also provide valuable scientific information (e.g. for the study of prognoses, harm or aethiology), but they usually carry less

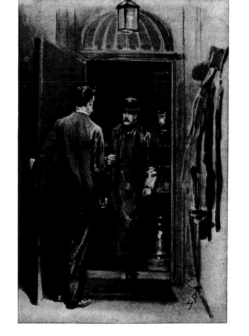

It didn't escape my notice. I began to smell a rat. You know the feeling, Mr Sherlock Holmes, when you come upon the right scent – a kind of thrill in your nerves.
Inspector Gregson in *A Study in Scarlet.*

weight than an RCT. There are different types of observational studies and, in general, the further the study design departs from that of the RCT the less it protects against bias and the weaker the evidence.

The *hierarchy of evidence* in scientific investigations can be seen from the table below:

	Study design		
	---	---	---
Type of study	**Randomized**	**Prospective**	**Control/comparison group**
RCT	√	√	√
Non-randomized study with contemporary or historical controls	–	√	√
Cohort study	–	√ / –	√
Case–control study	–	– / √	√
Cross-sectional study	–	–	√
Study with consecutive cases	–	– / √	–
Case report	–	–	–

The Randomized Control Trial (RCT)

The RCT is the type of study that has the highest potential for determining the effects of specific actions and treatments. In an RCT, a population of individuals is allocated to two or more groups. One group is allocated to a control group (and receives the standard treatment or an ineffective treatment or substance: a placebo) while the other group make up the experiment group and receive the experimental treatment, the effects of which one wants to evaluate. All groups are followed up during a specified period of time and the predetermined outcome (e.g. mortality, myocardial infarction, blood concentration) is analysed. The allocation/randomization is carried out so as to render the groups comparable. In the ideal instance, the groups should be the same apart from the experimental intervention or treatment under study. Of course, in practice, it is impossible to study absolutely identical groups of patients who are exposed to exactly the same conditions during the trial period apart from the experimental intervention/treatment. As a consequence, a critical evaluation of the methods and results is necessary.

Observational studies

A *cohort study* is an observational study in which the individuals are grouped according to their having previously been exposed, or not exposed, to some form of phenomenon and are then followed over time. A *cohort* is a group of patients having a number of characteristics in common. (The name stems from the Latin *cohors*: tenth part of a legion in the ancient Roman armies.) Synonymous terms for cohort studies are longitudinal, prospective and incidence studies. The design of cohort studies can be either prospective or retrospective (historical).

In *case–control studies*, patients with a certain outcome are compared with patients not having the outcome for the purpose of determining factors that might have caused the differences between the groups.

A *cross-sectional study* involves a defined group of patients examined at a specific point in time or time interval. Cross-sectional studies have the disadvantage of not providing direct evidence of the sequence of events and are subject to measurement and confounding biases.

A *study with consecutive cases (case series)* and *case reports* are descriptions of a group of patients or an individual patient, respectively, with the intention to inform about a new or not widely recognized aspect of a disease or therapy.

The *level of evidence* refers to the validity of an individual study based on an assessment of its study design:

Graded level of evidence	Signification	Background
A	Strong scientific evidence	Evidence obtained from meta-analyses, systematic reviews or large, well-made RCTs
B	Moderate evidence studies or cross-sectional studies, case–control studies	Evidence obtained from small or not optimally conducted randomized studies or from studies without randomization (cohort studies)
C	Weak evidence	Expert opinions, consensus reports, case reports and other descriptive studies
D	Scientific evidence lacking	No studies with satisfactory quality are available

The hierarchy is not absolute, however. If, for instance, there is a large, clear-cut, therapeutic effect, the value of an observational study may be higher than that of many RCTs. Some examples of this are observational studies reporting benefits of prosthetic surgery in osteoarthrosis of the hip, surgical drainage of abscesses and insulin therapy in diabetic ketoacidosis.

In most cases, observational studies accurately predict the findings of subsequent RCTs, but there are examples where large discrepancies have been noted. A randomized trial may not always be feasible or, in some circumstances, may not be the optimal study design. Observational studies may sometimes provide more reliable information, e.g. when reporting rare adverse effects and case studies may yield high-quality evidence for uncommon disorders and for complication rates in interventional procedures or surgery.

Some authorities claim that the quality of a scientific article can be judged to a certain extent by where it was published. This is based on the fact that the more prestigious journals with a wide circulation receive many manuscripts for review and that such journals usually have in place a rigorous review procedure. This is, however, a simplified approach: every scientific publication must be judged on its own merits. The so-called *impact factor* (IF) of a journal refers to the frequency with which its articles are cited in articles in other journals. The higher the IF, the more prestigious the journal. Only some 20% of all journals have an IF of over 2, so that an IF of over 2 or 3 may be classified as high.

Examples of clinical journals with a high IF (January 2006) are as follows:

Journal	IF
New England Journal of Medicine	39
Journal of American Medical Association	25
The Lancet	22
Gastroenterology	13
Circulation	13
Journal of Clinical Oncology	10
Diabetes	9
American Journal of Psychiatry	8
British Medical Journal	7
Gut	6
European Heart Journal	6
Annals of Surgery	6
Journal of Clinical Endocrinology and Metabolism	6
Pediatrics	4

PubMed comprises the search term AIM (*Abridged Index Medicus*), which enables searches in 120 selected so-called core clinical journals, i.e. in some of the most important and most influential clinical journals in existence. Among the publications included in AIM are all clinical journals with a high IF. If you, for example, conduct a PubMed search on Parkinson's disease with AIM, your search will be limited to these well-reputed journals. This can be very useful if you are looking for, let us say, a review article.

Evaluation of the scientific quality

A scientific study stands and falls with its quality. This section deals with how to pose specific questions for the evaluation of the scientific value of an article. It is easy to feel overwhelmed when confronted with a scientific report. Many studies are complex and detailed and you may feel insecure about the study design or about the way the statistical analysis has been carried out. In reality, it does not have to be overly difficult to critically assess medical articles since the process may be systematized by use of standardized critical appraisal tools. Standard critical appraisal tools have been developed to assess the quality of research reports. More than 100 such appraisal tools are available, but only a

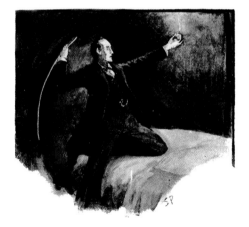

Circumstantial evidence is a very tricky thing. It may point very straight to one thing, but if you shift your own point of view a little, you may find it pointing in an equally uncompromising manner to something entirely different.

Sherlock Holmes in *The Boscombe Valley Mystery.*

few have documented evidence of the validity of their items or the reliability of their use [8]. Unfortunately, there is considerable variation in their intent, components and construction and there is no consensus regarding the "gold standard" tool for critical appraisal of research reports.

The aim of critical appraisal tools is to provide analytical evaluations of study quality in order to minimize bias and it is important for consumers of research to ascertain whether the results can be believed and transferred to clinical practice.

In this section we shall use a simplified critical appraisal tool for quality assessment based on a number of questions:

Question	Elicits answers concerning
Why?	The aim
In what way?	Design and execution
How good?	Quality
How big?	Effect
How sure?	Reliability
So what?	Relevance/significance

The majority of critical appraisal tools are research design-specific and contain items that address methodological issues that are unique to the study design. At present there is no validated generic critical appraisal tool so each research design needs to be evaluated by specific items. Thus, there are specific evaluation tools for experimental, diagnostic, observational and qualitative studies, as well as for systematic reviews/meta-analyses [8]. Widely used critical appraisal tools are CONSORT for RCTs (therapy studies), STARD (Standard for Reporting of Diagnostic Accuracy) for diagnostic tests and QUORUM for meta-analyses. These tools are available at **www.consort-statement.org**

Some critical appraisal tools (e.g. CONSORT) have a structure based on the preferred format for reporting research communications (Title, Abstract, Introduction, Methods, Results and Discussion). This format is helpful both for readers assessing the content and for trialists when planning or writing up clinical studies. Other appraisal tools focus on the key aspects of quality. One such tool used by the Cochrane Collaboration comprises 11 key items for quality assessment [9]:

- Study aims and justification
- Methodology used
- Sample selection
- Method of randomization and allocation blinding

- Attrition: response and drop-out rates
- Blinding
- Outcome measure
- Intervention
- Method of data analysis
- Potential sources of bias
- External validity.

The AGREE instrument is an appraisal tool designed to help guideline developers and users assess the methodological quality of Clinical Practice Guidelines. It is available from **www.agreecollaboration.org**

On the following pages, we shall critically appraise four different types of study with the aid of posed questions, namely:
- Studies concerning therapy (pp. 44–51)
- Studies concerning diagnostic tests (pp. 51–60)
- Systematic reviews/meta-analysis (pp. 60–64)
- Clinical Practice Guidelines (pp. 64–65).

When you appraise a study you must consider whether you can answer "Yes", "Not clear" or "No" to the posed questions. The more the "No" responses, the less valuable the study.

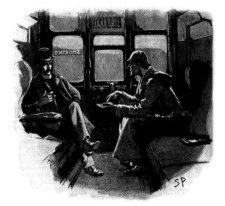

– And what do you think of it all, Watson? Asked Sherlock Holmes.
– It seems to me to be a most dark and sinister business.
– Dark enough and sinister enough.
Holmes and Watson in *The Adventure of the Speckled Band.*

Critical appraisal of therapy studies

The ACP Journal Club has three explicit criteria for scientific merit, which all studies of therapy must fulfil to be considered for assessment:
- Random allocation of participants to comparison groups
- Follow up of at least 80% of those entering the investigation
- Outcome measure of known or probable clinical importance.

These criteria can be considered to represent a minimum level of scientific merit for potentially useful clinical studies.

Ask the following questions:

Why? (The aim)
Question 1: Is the scientific question (or problem) clearly stated?
The type of patients studied, the intervention affected and the outcome investigated should already be evident from the summary of, or introduction to, the article.

In what way? (Design and execution)
Question 2: What type of study is it? Have the investigators used the right experimental design to find the answer to their question? Were the patients randomized?

An RCT reduces the risk of systematic errors (bias) owing to differences between the patients who receive the treatment under study and those who do not. Other experimental designs, e.g. cohort, case-control or cross-sectional studies, can also produce valuable results, but their value is usually lower than that of an RCT.

Question 3: Who are the patients? Is the patient population clearly described and what are the inclusion and exclusion criteria?

Every study addresses an issue relevant to some population with the condition of interest. Investigators restrict this population by using eligibility criteria. Typical selection criteria may relate to age, sex, clinical diagnosis and co-morbid conditions; exclusion criteria are often used to ensure patient safety. Of particular importance is the method of recruitment, such as by referral or self-selection (e.g. through advertisements).

How good? (Quality)
Question 4: Is the study large enough or does it include just a few events or observations? Is the presented data informative or not? Are the results for all patients included in the study reported?

If the drop-out rate is high, it will reduce the value of the study.

Are results are based on the *intention-to-treat* principle, i.e. were all patients in the final analysis of the study assigned to the group to which they were initially allocated? If they were not, the true effect may have been concealed. The significance of the analysis based on the intention-to-treat principle can be illustrated by the following Sherlock Holmes' episode.

EXAMPLE

In *The Adventure of the Empty House*, Holmes requested help from Scotland Yard to apprehend a man suspected of murdering Mr Ronald Adair. Inspectors Lestrade and Gregson decided to take five constables each with them to Baker Street. But what is the quickest way to get from Scotland Yard to Baker Street? Lestrade chose a horse and carriage, Gregson the recently built London Underground. Lestrade's party set off in three carriages. Gregson and his men took the Underground from Charing Cross to the Baker Street Underground Railway Station.

The results were as follows:

Lestrade and company: One carriage arrived without a problem in 30 min.

The second carriage lost a wheel and the occupants were therefore obliged to take the Underground. They arrived after 60 min.

The third carriage was stopped on the way by a fire in Regent Street and therefore never got to Baker Street.

Mean travel time for Lestrade and his men turned out to be 45 min (30 min, $n = 2$; 60 min, $n = 2$ and drop-outs, $n = 2$).

Gregson and company: Running smoothly, the Underground got all the policemen there in 40 min.

If we disregard the failures with two of Lestrade's carriages, the one carriage transport was the fastest: the only carriage that got there made the trip in 30 min. The underground took 40 min for Gregson's men and 60 min for two of Lestrade's men.

However, if an analysis is performed according to the intention-to-treat principle, the Underground is found to be both faster and better (mean travel time, 40 min, $n = 6$) than the horse and carriage (mean travel time, 45 min, $n = 4$). It is true that some of the men allocated to the horse and carriage reached their destination after 30 min, but two men were delayed and another two did not arrive at all.

Question 5: Was the treatment blinded?

In controlled trials, the term *blinding* refers to keeping study participants, health care providers and those collecting and analyzing clinical data unaware of the assigned intervention so that they will not be influenced by that knowledge.

Blinding of patients is important because knowledge of the group assignment may influence responses to treatment. Blinding should not be confused with *allocation concealment*, which seeks to prevent bias by protecting the assignment sequence before and until allocation. In contrast, blinding seeks to prevent performance bias (by patients or health care providers) and assignment bias (by those evaluating outcomes).

Question 6: Were the groups similar from the beginning?

If there were differences at baseline with regard to important demographic (e.g. age, gender) or clinical characteristics (diagnosis, etc.), the groups were not comparable.

Question 7: Did the groups receive similar treatments apart from the experimental treatment or intervention? If there were other circumstances, e.g. different observation periods, this may have influenced the results.

How big? (Effect)

Question 8: How big an effect did the treatment have?

The following concepts are important for the quantification of observed differences: *relative risk* (RR), *relative risk reduction* (RRR), *absolute risk reduction* (ARR), *numbers-needed-to-treat* (NNT) and *odds ratio* (OR). The following narrative can illustrate the meanings of these terms.

EXAMPLE

In *The Adventure of the Speckled Band*, Grimesby Roylott dies after being bitten by an Indian swamp snake, the most poisonous snake in India, according to Watson. Watson might have been able to save Roylott's life if antivenom serum had been available. However, no antiserum existed at the time in question and Watson may have hesitated anyway to administer anti-snakebite serum because of the risk of excessively serious side-effects.

In a randomized study conducted in Sri Lanka, the investigators studied the possibility of reducing allergic reactions to antivenom serum by prophylactic subcutaneous injection of adrenaline [10]. One hundred and five snake-bitten subjects were studied, 56 of whom received adrenaline and 49 placebo. Allergic reactions to antivenom serum were observed in 6 patients (11%) in the adrenaline group and in 21 patients (43%) in the placebo group. Is this a big effect of treatment?

The results can be analysed with the aid of a 2 × 2 table:

	Outcome		
	Event	**Non-event**	**Sum**
Experiment group	a	b	$a + b$
Control group	c	d	$c + d$

Risk in the experimental group = $a / (a + b)$
Risk in the control group = $c / (c + d)$
Relative risk (RR) = $[a / (a + b)] / [c / (c + d)]$
Relative risk reduction (RRR) = $[c / (c + d) - a / (a + b)] / [c / (c + d)]$
Absolute risk reduction (ARR) = $[c / (c + d)] - [a / (a + b)]$
Numbers-needed-to-treat (NNT) = $1 / ARR$
Odds in experiment group = a / b
Odds in control group = c / d
Odds ratio (OR) = $(a / b) / (c / d)$

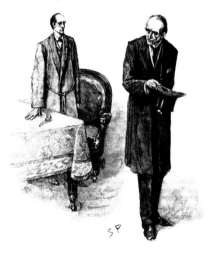

Though most of the facts were familiar to me, I had not sufficiently appreciated their relative importance, nor their connection to each other.
Watson in *Silver Blaze*.

The effect of prophylactic adrenaline on allergic reactions to antivenom serum can be expressed in the following manner:

	Outcome		
	Allergic reaction	**No allergic reaction**	**Sum**
Adrenaline prophylaxis	$a = 6$	$b = 50$	$a + b = 56$
Placebo	$c = 21$	$d = 28$	$c + d = 49$

RR, RRR, NNT and OR can be calculated using the above formulae, but they can also be worked out together with the 95% confidence interval (CI) by using one of the many excellent spreadsheets (calculating programs) available on the Web (see p. 81). Go to **www.healthcare.ubc.ca**, → Links, → Calculators, → Clinical significance calculator. You will discover the following:

RR = 0.25 (0.11–0.57; 95% CI)
RR indicates that the risk of having an allergic reaction after adrenaline is one fourth of the risk occurring if adrenaline is not given for prophylaxis. Thus RR does not describe the absolute but rather the relative benefit. A significant RR > 2 (or <0.5) may be considered to be strong and RR > 10 (or RR < 0.2) very strong evidence of association.

RRR = 75% (43–89; 95% CI)
This shows that an adrenaline injection reduces the risk of an allergic reaction by 75% compared with placebo. The higher the RRR, the more effective the treatment.

ARR = 32% (16–48; 95% CI)
Adrenaline gave rise to an absolute decrease in the proportion of allergic reactions by 32%. ARR describes both the underlying risk in the control group and the reduced risk that the experimental treatment can bring about. ARR has a clear clinical significance and is therefore an important concept that can be applied in many clinical situations.

NNT = 3 (2–6; 95% CI)
If we treat three patients with adrenaline, one case of allergic reaction will be prevented. NNT is a useful concept because it combines statistical and clinical information in a readily comprehensible manner.

OR = 0.16 (0.05–0.49; 95% CI)
OR < 1 indicates a reduced risk, OR = 1 the same risk and OR > 1 an increased risk. OR is used in, for instance, retrospective studies, cross-sectional

studies and meta-analyses (p. 60ff.) where the aim is to describe relationships rather than exact differences.

Thus the effect of treatment can be described by calculations of different risk measurements or in terms of odds. The question is, then, if we should be impressed by a new treatment with NNT = 3?

At **www.cebm.utoronto.ca/glossary/nnts.htm** you will find NNT listings for a large number of studies. NNT < 10 can be considered to be a relatively large effect. Our NNT = 3 for adrenaline prophylaxis against allergic reactions to antivenom serum must therefore be regarded as a large prophylactic effect. A small effect of treatment (with high NNT) can, however, sometimes be clinically important in serious outcomes (e.g. stroke, death) while a large effect of treatment (with low NNT) may be clinically unimportant in less serious outcomes. So NNT should not be judged only in terms of the numerical value, but clinical factors must also be considered. It is important in all assessments of risk and odds to specify the follow-up time as these parameters may look different from a perspective of, say, 5 or 15 years.

If a treatment is harmful so that the success rate is less than that on the control treatment, the NNT will be negative. This number is then called the *numbers-needed to-harm* (NNH).

How sure? (Reliability)

Question 9: How sure can you be of the observed effect of treatment?

For each outcome, study results should be reported as a summary of the outcome in each group together with the contrast between the groups, known as the effect size. Some useful concepts here are *statistical significance*, the *p-value* and *Confidence Interval (CI)*.

The *p*-value is a measure of probability. One proceeds from a null hypothesis (the hypothesis that no effect or difference exists). If an effect or difference is determined (i.e. the null hypothesis is rejected), the *p*-value indicates the probability that the effect or difference may be due to chance. $p < 0.05$ indicates that the probability of the effect or difference being due to chance is less than 5%. When *p* is found to be 0.05 or lower, the effect or difference is said to be statistically significant.

The CI describes the interval within which the true value probably lies. In most cases, the 95% CI is given, which means that the true value will range between the stated values with a 95% probability. If the stated CI includes the value at which "no difference is present" (i.e. the events in the experiment group and the control group are the same), there is no statistical significance. If RR = 0.8 and the 95% CI is 0.6–1.1, there is no statistical significance because CI includes 1.0 (where RR is the same for the experiment group and the control group). If, on the other hand, RR = 0.6 and the 95% CI is 0.4–0.9, there is a statistical significance as CI does not pass through 1.0.

Two types of errors may occur in statistical calculations. A *type I error* (*alpha error*) occurs when a study finds a difference between the groups when there actually is none, i.e. a false-positive result. This corresponds to the situation when a court of law convicts an innocent person.

A *type II error* (*beta error*) occurs when no difference is found when a difference actually exists, i.e. a false-negative result. The court acquits a person who has committed a crime.

So what? (Relevance/clinical significance)

Question 10: Can the results be utilized in the care of my patients?

One of the first considerations is whether or not your patient really resembles the patients included in the study. Perhaps the study population had a more advanced form of the disease than your patient has? Perhaps your patient also has other diseases that did not occur in the study patients?

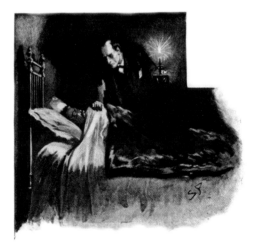

Holmes shook his head like a man who is far from being satisfied.
– These are very deep waters.
Sherlock Holmes in *The Adventure of the Speckled Band.*

External validity, also called generalizability or applicability, is the extent to which the results of a study can be generalized to other circumstances.

There are a number of other considerations (potential benefit and harm, patients' values and preferences) that need to be addressed before the results of a trial can be applied to individual patients. These aspects are discussed further in Step 4 (p. 69ff.).

Critical appraisal of diagnostic tests

The most frequently conducted clinical trials pertain to treatment strategies (therapy). The second most usual ones deal with problems related to confirming (or ruling out) disease in symptomatic patients (diagnostic tests) or in individuals without symptoms (screening). A diagnostic test is generally considered to be a laboratory test that produces a result in the form of a numerical value. However, the definition can also be widened to include other forms of tests or examinations and evaluate them in respect of their ability to distinguish between subjects who have a disease and those who do not. The result of a test can be described in terms of, for instance, the absence or presence of a symptom or a clinical sign or an examined radiograph or histopathological specimen, as well as a laboratory test result.

To reach a diagnosis is an imperfect process which is based on probabilities rather than on absolute confidence in the correct diagnosis. A perfect diagnostic test has 100% sensitivity (i.e. all sick subjects show a positive test result) and 100% specificity (i.e. all well subjects show a negative test result). In practice, however, there are no diagnostic tests with that degree of reliability. We must therefore learn to deal with the limitations that all diagnostic tests have. Some important terms for expressing the usefulness of a test are *sensitivity*, *specificity*, *predictive value (PV)* and *likelihood ratio (LR)*.

Odds and probabilities

Sensitivity, specificity and PV are measures of probabilities and the LR is a measure of odds. The concepts of probability and odds contain the same information but they describe it differently.

Probability is the proportion of patients in whom a particular characteristic (e.g. a positive test result) is present.

Odds are the ratio between two probabilities: the probability of an event to that of a non-event (1 − probability of the event).

$$\text{Odds} = \frac{\text{Probability}}{1 - \text{Probability}}$$

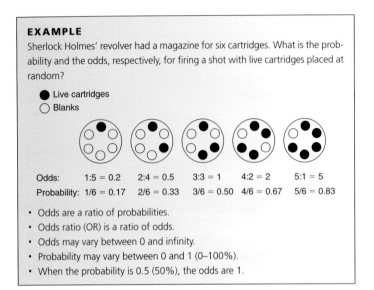

EXAMPLE

Sherlock Holmes' revolver had a magazine for six cartridges. What is the probability and the odds, respectively, for firing a shot with live cartridges placed at random?

● Live cartridges
○ Blanks

Odds: 1:5 = 0.2   2:4 = 0.5   3:3 = 1   4:2 = 2   5:1 = 5
Probability: 1/6 = 0.17   2/6 = 0.33   3/6 = 0.50 4/6 = 0.67 5/6 = 0.83

- Odds are a ratio of probabilities.
- Odds ratio (OR) is a ratio of odds.
- Odds may vary between 0 and infinity.
- Probability may vary between 0 and 1 (0–100%).
- When the probability is 0.5 (50%), the odds are 1.

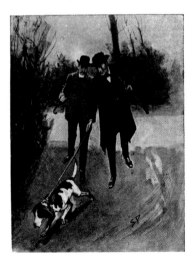

What one man can invent, another can discover.
Sherlock Holmes in *The Adventure of the Dancing Men.*

Let us illustrate the problem and how the shortcomings of diagnostic tests can be described and quantified by means of an example from the world of Sherlock Holmes.

EXAMPLE

The detective work done by Inspector Lestrade at Scotland Yard resulted in 10 people being put on trial, charged with murder. Seven of them were indeed real murderers, but three of them had not committed murder. (Sherlock Holmes was not particularly impressed by Lestrade's detective work.) The ruling of the court was as follows:

- Four murderers were convicted of murder.
- Three murderers were acquitted.
- One innocent person was convicted of murder.
- Two innocent persons were acquitted.

The results can be presented in a 2 × 2 table. Note that the true distribution (which ones are really murderers and which ones are innocent) is presented in the vertical cells. The ruling of the court (which does not necessarily reflect the truth) is presented in horizontal cells.

	True distribution		
Court's ruling	**Murderer**	**Innocent**	**Totals**
Guilty = "Murderer"	4	1	5
Acquitted = "Innocent"	3	2	5
Totals	7	3	

The ruling of the court can be summarized as follows:
- Four of seven real murderers were convicted of murder. Sensitivity: $4/7 = 0.57 = 56\%$.
- Two of the three innocent persons were acquitted. Specificity: $2/3 = 0.67 = 67\%$.
- Three of the seven real murderers were acquitted.
- One of the three innocent persons was convicted.
- Six of the ten accused persons had a just conviction.

A 2 × 2 table is used to assess diagnostic tests in medicine. The values obtained with a new test method are compared with those obtained with the best currently available one (the reference method). The reference method values are presented vertically in the table and the new method's values horizontally.

Results of the new test	Reference method			
	Presence of disease	Absence of disease	Totals	
Positive test	a = true-positive	b = false-positive	$a + b$ →	$PV+ = \dfrac{a}{a + b}$
Negative test	c = false-negative	d = true-negative	$c + d$ →	$PV- = \dfrac{d}{c + d}$
Totals	$a + c$ ↓ $Se = \dfrac{a}{a + c}$	$b + d$ ↓ $Sp = \dfrac{d}{b + d}$	$a + b + c + d$	

PV+ = Positive predictive value; PV− = Negative predictive value;
Se = Sensitivity; Sp = Specificity

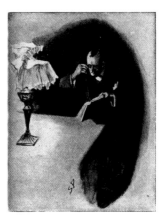

Singularity is almost invariably a clue. The more featureless and commonplace a crime is, the more difficult it is to bring home.
Sherlock Holmes in *The Boscombe Valley Mystery.*

Term	Meaning	Calculation
Sensitivity	To what extent can a test demonstrate disease?	$a / (a + c)$
Specificity	To what extent can a test rule out disease?	$d / (b + d)$
Prevalence	The fundamental risk of disease in a particular population	$(a + c) / (a + b + c + d)$
PV+	How high is the *probability* for a disease in a person with a positive test result?	$a / (a + b)$
PV−	How high is the *probability* for not having a disease in a person with a negative test result?	$d / (c + d)$
LR for a positive test result (LR+)	How high are the *odds* for a positive test result in a sick person in relation to a positive test result in a well person?	Sensitivity / (1 − Specificity)
LR for a negative test result (LR−)	How high are the *odds* for a negative test result in a sick person in relation to a negative test result in a well person?	(1 − Sensitivity) / Specificity

A good test produces results in which the majority of the measurements are true-positive ("*a*" in the above table) or true-negative ("*d*"). Very few tests are, however, perfect, so you will get a certain proportion of false-positive ("*b*") and false-negative ("*c*") results. Sensitivity and specificity are important terms that can be applied to different types of test.

Sensitivity indicates how many of the subjects who are really ill test positive for the illness. In other words, how good is the test at demonstrating illness in individuals who are really ill?

Specificity indicates how many of the subjects who are really healthy test negative for the illness. In other words, how good is the test at ruling out illness in individuals who are actually healthy.

The sensitivity and specificity of a test can be changed if the limits are changed. Increasing the sensitivity leads to an increase in the number of true-positives ("*a*"). But, in practice, this also entails an increase in the number of false-positives "*b*", i.e. the specificity decreases.

The higher the sensitivity of a test, the surer you can be that a negative result rules out the diagnosis (a high sensitivity yields few false-negative results). Remember: **SnNout** = when a test has a high **Sen**sitivity, a **N**egative result rules **out** the diagnosis.

The higher the specificity of a test, the surer you can be that a positive test result rules in the diagnosis. Remember: **SpPin** = when a test has a high **Sp**ecificity, a **P**ositive result rules **in** the diagnosis [1].

It is true that calculations of the sensitivity and specificity of a test give some idea of its strength, but this does not make it possible to calculate the probablility or the odds for demonstrating disease in a particular patient. If the sensitivity and specificity are known, it is possible to calculate the PV or the LR.

The PV+ is the probablility of disease in a person with a positive (abnormal) test result. The PV− is the probability of not having the disease in a person with a negative (normal) test result. PV+ = 0.80 indicates that in a person with a positive test result, the probability that the person has the disease is 80% (with a 20% probability of not having the disease).

The PV can be calculated if the test's sensitivity and specificity are known, but the PV is also dependent on the prevalence of the disease in the population being tested. This is a drawback since you would like to use a test that is dependent only on its discriminating capacity to diagnose the particular disease, irrespective of the prevalence of the disease in the population. If the prevalence is high in the population (higher than 2–5%), the calculation of the PV can be meaningful, but in populations where the prevalence of the disease is low, the concept of PV becomes meaningless (as the prevalence approaches zero the PV+ also approaches zero).

A concept which is more clinically useful for assessing the validity of a test stems from the likelihood concept (Bayes theorem). LR is calculated from the sensitivity and specificity of a test and has the advantage of being independent of the prevalence of the disease. LR tells us the extent (the odds) to which we may assume that a certain test result is true.

A test's LR+ is calculated as:

$$LR+ = \frac{\text{Probability of a positive test result in a person with the disease}}{\text{Probability of a positive test result in a person without the disease}} = \frac{\text{Sensitivity}}{1 - \text{Specificity}}$$

Since LR is a measure of the odds, an LR value of 1 means that the test lacks a discriminating capability.

LR for a positive test result (LR+) shows how much the odds increase for the presence of disease in cases with a positive test result. The best test for establishing the presence of disease is the one that has the highest odds in cases with a positive test result and an LR+ greater than 10 is usually considered to rule in a particular diagnosis.

When a test result is negative, LR− can be calculated in a corresponding manner: the probability of a negative test result in a person with the disease divided by the probability of a negative test result in a non-diseased person ((1 − sensitivity) / specificity). LR for a negative test result (LR−) shows how much the odds decrease for the presence of disease in cases with a negative test result. The best test to rule out disease has the lowest odds in cases with a negative test result and an LR− smaller than 0.1, means in practice that a particular diagnosis can be ruled out.

The strength of different LRs to change the likelihood of the presence of disease is indicated below (LR > 1 increases the likelihood, LR < 1 decreases the likelihood of the presence of the disease in question):

LR	Meaning
>10	Very large, often conclusive, increase
5–10	Moderate increase
2–5	Small increase
1–2	Minimal increase
1	No change
0.5–1.0	Small decrease
0.1–0.2	Moderate decrease
<0.1	Very large, often conclusive, decrease

In order to be able to judge the potential worth of a test, it is necessary to know the frequency of the disease/symptom in the population (the *prevalence*): the *pre-test probability* (i.e. what we believed before we used the test). In addition, we must take account of information about the ability of the test to discriminate, preferably expressed as LR. With the aid of the pre-test probably and LR, we can calculate the *post-test probability*. The calculations are rather complicated so that the simplest solution is to use a Web-based calculator (Bayes calculator, see p. 81) for this purpose.

EXAMPLE

Let us return to the courtroom example from the world of Sherlock Holmes and characterize the ruling of the court (the reliability of the test method) and what consequences it has regarding the possibility of judging real murderers correctly (post-test probability):

You know the following from the above account (p. 53ff.):
Sensitivity = 57% = 0.57
Specificity = 67% = 0.67
Pre-test probability (= prevalence of "true" murderers) = 7/10 = 0.70

You will now use a Web-based spreadsheet (see p. 79), e.g. **www.healthcare.ubc.ca**, go to Links → Calculators → Bayesean calculator and you will find the following:
LR+ = 1.72
Post-test probability = 0.80 = 80%

The value for LR+ is 1.72 and, according to the above table, this means that the test gives the lowest possible probability (i.e. a "minimal increase") of a positive outcome, i.e. of convicting murderers of murder. The probability of "true" murderers being justly convicted is 80%.

Proceeding from the questions posed on p. 42, we shall now make a critical appraisal of a diagnostic study.

The ACP Journal Club appraisal protocol states that studies of diagnosis should meet the following basic criteria for quality:

- Inclusion of a spectrum of participants, some but not all of whom have the disorder of interest.
- Objective diagnostic ("gold") standard or current clinical standard for diagnosis.
- Each participant must have both the new and some form of diagnostic standard.
- Interpretation of the diagnostic standard without any knowledge of the test result.
- Interpretation of test without any knowledge of the diagnostic standard result.

Ask the following questions:

Why? (The aim)
Question 1: Is the scientific problem clearly stated?

The study should be focused on a diagnostic problem of clinical significance. Is the new test more reliable? Cheaper?

In what way? (Design and execution)
Question 2: Is the population studied clearly defined and is it relevant to the test being evaluated?

How does the gender and age distribution look?

The included patients should be ones with respectively mild and advanced disease, as well as treated and untreated ones, and also include some with other diseases that often come into differential diagnostic consideration.

Question 3: Is the test being evaluated comparable to the best available test method ("the gold standard") and was blinding carried out in the appraisal?

Each individual must have been tested with both the new diagnostic test and the one currently considered to be the best. In certain cases, the standard test may be of an entirely different type (a radiological method, explorative surgery, biopsy, etc.) from the new test which is to be evaluated.

How good? (Quality)
Question 4: What are the estimates of diagnostic accuracy and measures of statistical uncertainty (e.g. 95% CI)? What are the estimates of variability of diagnostic accuracy between subgroups of patients or centres? Is the reproducibility of the test known?

Ideally, if the test is repeated several times on the same individual(s) or if the test results are analysed by different investigators, the values obtained should be the same. One way to express reproducibility is to calculate the *coefficient of variation* (CV):

$CV = (SD / mean) \times 100$, where SD is the standard deviation.

How sure? (Reliability)
Question 5: How reliable are tests designed to diagnose or, conversely, rule out disease?

The key concepts here are the sensitivity of the new test, which reflects its ability to diagnose disease in sick subjects, and its specificity, which reflects its ability to rule out disease in healthy subjects. LR describes the odds for a specific test result being true. The calculations are performed as shown above (p. 55ff.).

So what? (Relevance/significance)

Question 6: Are the results applicable to my patients and do they change my treatment strategies?

You must decide whether the new test has the potential for practical use in your clinic or whether it affects treatment strategies. This aspect is discussed later (p. 69ff.).

Critical appraisal of a systematic review/meta-analysis

A systematic review implies that one has collected all relevant information, critically appraised and summated the evidence in a specific subject area. In the collection of data, great importance is attached to obtaining all relevant information (both positive and negative results) from published and unpublished investigations. As a rule, use is made of a review "template" created in advance and upon which an assessment of the quality of the collected material is based. In as much as randomized trials are the most reliable studies, the greatest emphasis is placed on such trials. Original data can be used to effectuate a compilation of the results in order to increase the probability of demonstrating whether a difference really exists (increasing the power of the analysis).

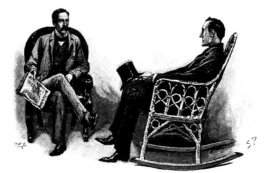

It is my business to know things. Perhaps I have trained myself to see what others overlook.
Sherlock Holmes in *A Case of Identity.*

In a meta-analysis, the results obtained are summarized by means of a statistical analysis of the included studies. In order to make different studies comparable in meta-analyses, use is often made of the OR (see also p. 46ff.). By the term odds is meant the relationship between the winnings and the stakes. OR expresses the odds for an experiment group showing positive or, conversely, negative effects of an intervention in relation to a control group. OR < 1 indicates a reduced risk, OR $= 1$ the same risk and OR > 1 an increased risk. The numerical value is an expression of the power of the ratio.

The figure below shows a typical presentation of the results of a meta-analysis investigating the effects of beta-carotene treatment on cardiac events.

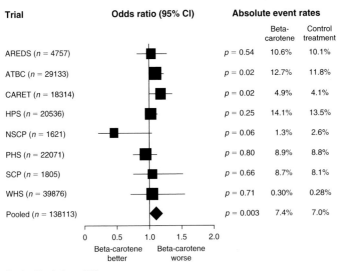

Breslow-Day test: $p = 0.32$

OR (95% CI) for total mortality among individuals treated with beta-carotene or control therapy (Ref. 6 [fig. 1], reproduced with the kind permission of Elsevier, The Lancet).

The figure is from the meta-analysis published by Vivekananthan et al. [6] in which the authors appraised the effect of antioxidants in patients with cardiovascular disease. OR and the 95% CI are indicated for the eight different individual studies and for all of them combined, the latter being represented by a diamond-shaped symbol. The figure shows that beta-carotene was associated with increased mortality in two of the studies (ATBC and CARET; $p = 0.003$). No statistically significant differences were observed in the other studies. The combined results show that beta-carotene increased mortality.

In the same way as we did with studies dealing with therapy or diagnostics, we will now pose questions to evaluate critically systematic reviews and meta-analyses.

The basic requirements for a systematic review to be considered to be of scientific value include:
- Strict criteria should have been used when choosing articles to be included (inclusion and exclusion criteria should have been specified) and regarding how the validity of the studies has been assessed.
- A comprehensive search process should have been undertaken in order to retrieve all relevant studies.

Why? (The aim)
Question 1: Is the clinical problem or question in the systematic review clearly stated and how well does it match your clinical problem?

In what way? (Design and execution)
Question 2: Is the article a meta-analysis (data statistically analysed) or a systematic review in the wider meaning of the term?

Question 3: How was the search for the articles conducted and was it extensive and exhaustive?

The information sources that were used should be stated in detail (e.g. databases, registers, personal files, agencies, hand-searching). Any restrictions should be stated (years considered, language of publication).

Studies which do not obtain statistically significant results have a tendency to remain unpublished, which can result in a publication bias. This means that the true effect of an intervention can be overrated in a systematic review. It should be clearly shown in the Method section how the articles were obtained and how the data were processed.

Question 4: How were the articles selected?

Selection criteria (population, intervention, outcome, study design) should be stated. The RCT forms the basis for all well-elaborated systematic reviews and meta-analyses. Strict inclusion criteria must have been employed.

How good? (Quality)

Question 5: Are the studies included mutually congruent?

The degree of heterogeneity can be calculated statistically. A rough estimate of the heterogeneity can also be made by seeing whether the CIs are fairly similar. How long are the "tails"?

Go back to the figure on p. 61. In that figure, the NSCP study seems to be quite different from the other studies: the mean value is quite different and the "tails" are quite long (broad CIs). Furthermore, the NSCP study is the smallest of the studies included in this meta-analysis. Thus the NSCP study differ from the others and the validity of this study may be questioned. It is, however, important not to exclude studies that differ from the others – if they meet the inclusion criteria.

Question 6: Is the summary based on a synthesis that satisfies the predefined inclusion criteria?

One should be observant of any subgroup analyses that may have been performed. The relevance of subgroup analyses increases if an hypothesis was proposed before the study was made, if the subgroup was large and if large and strong significant differences were found between the subgroups.

How big? (Effect)

Question 7: How big is the effect of treatment?

When it comes to systematic reviews the procedure followed to include individual studies is of a qualitative nature, which means that the results cannot be ascertained or presented numerically. Thus, the conclusion is based to a certain extent on a subjective assessment by the reviewers.

The procedure in a meta-analysis, on the other hand, involves the use of statistical methods to combine and summarize data from the available studies quantitatively. Thus a meta-analysis can ascertain the magnitude of an effect in numerical terms. In certain cases, it is also possible in meta-analyses to demonstrate by use of subgroup analyses new and previously unknown relationships.

How sure? (Reliability)

Question 8: How reliable is the result?

The result is dependent on whether or not all valid information has been included in the analyses. The search must have been made in different databases and include studies published in different languages (not only English). The search should have also been performed in areas beyond the conventional medical databases and include doctoral theses, pharmaceutical reports, unpublished studies, etc. The procedure for compiling, examining and evaluating the information obtained should also be followed rigorously. A well-performed meta-analysis including several well-conducted RCTs has a high degree of reliability (Evidence Level Grade A, p. 39).

So what? (Relevance/significance)

Question 9: How well do the patients on which the systematic review was based match your patient (diagnosis, age, gender, etc.)?

Question 10: Did the systematic review consider all clinically important aspects?

Many systematic reviews do not consider side-effects or such practical aspects as follow-up requirements. Costs must also be taken into consideration before the results can be applied in the daily clinical practice. Have the benefits been weighed against the risks and costs?

Critical appraisal of Clinical Practice Guidelines

Clinical Practice Guidelines consist of treatment recommendations for common clinical problems. Practice guidelines have always evoked strong feelings. Administrators and politicians are often strong advocates of practice guidelines for reasons of cost containment while health practitioners usually are more sceptical. The advocates often bring up considerations pertaining to fairness and uniform and standardized treatment strategies as important aspects. Sceptics feel that the practice guidelines do not take into consideration the individual patient's needs and tend to lead to mediocre rather than optimal care. The influence of the individual caregiver is also considered to be reduced. Sceptics also think that treatment routines developed on the national level may not be relevant on the local level.

During the last few years, a very large number of practice guidelines have been developed by the authorities, caregivers and specialist associations; in part as a means to increase the cost-effectiveness of health care. Clinical Practice Guidelines have become popular because they are concise and have an instructive make-up, but the scientific foundation varies very considerably. Many Clinical Practice Guidelines combine the results of clinical studies of varying quality with expert opinions. It is therefore important to gain insight into the quality of the specific guidelines.

Begin by checking which persons or organizations are behind the practice guideline. Is it an academic organization, a government authority, a sub-speciality interest group, or is there a commercial background? Who is the deliverer, what is the purpose and who financed the development of the programme? When was the programme updated the last time? What procedure was followed when developing it? How rigorous was the appraisal? Has evidence of harm been assessed and has reference to this been made?

The same type of appraisal can be made as in the case of systematic reviews and meta-analyses (p. 60). However, the concise, practical design of the guidelines is often an obstacle to critical appraisal. Clinical Practice Guidelines can be instructive and useful, but one must bear in mind their shortcomings, sometimes question their recommendations and, when necessary, make adjustments. After all, guidelines are only *guidelines* and not rigid directives for therapeutic interventions.

Why? (The aim)
Clinical Practice Guidelines may serve several purposes: to provide guidance in health care matters, reduce variations in care procedures, increase the quality of care, give guidance for resource allocation (cost containment), and/or promote training and education by means of updated literature reviews. A good Clinical Practice Guideline should be applicable to a clearly defined patient population and comprise all diagnostic and therapeutic aspects of the disease in question.

In what way? (Design and execution)
The expected outcome when the recommendations are followed should be stated and should be *clinically* important (e.g. influencing morbidity or mortality) rather than merely affecting *surrogate* parameters (e.g. laboratory test values, blood pressure, bone density).

How good? (Quality)
How was the guideline produced and what is the scientific basis for the recommendations (Evidence Level Grades A, B, C, D)? Is the description current and updated?

So what? (Relevance/significance)
Is the practice guideline applicable to my patient's disease and would its application have positive consequences for my patient? What does my patient think? Different guidelines apply to a greater or lesser extent to different institutions. Guidelines applicable to an academic tertiary referral centre may not be applicable to a small county hospital or in primary care.

Quality of evidence

The final step in your review of the information at hand is the grading of the quality of the evidence. This involves a general assessment based on the level of evidence (p. 39) and on the result of your critical appraisal. Quality is the extent to which the identified studies minimize the opportunity for bias and is synonymous with the concept of validity. Various organizations have presented models for formalizing the process of making judgements about the quality of evidence in order to prevent errors, facilitate critical appraisal and improve the communication of information. The GRADE Working Group recommends the following system for grading the quality of evidence [7]:

Grade of quality	Meaning
High	Further research is very unlikely to change the estimate of effect
Moderate	Further research is likely to change the estimate of effect
Low	Further research is very likely to change the estimate
Very low	Any estimate of effect is very uncertain

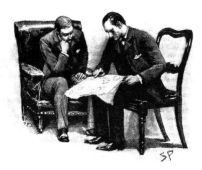

While the individual man is an insoluble puzzle, in the aggregate he becomes a mathematical certainty. You can, for example, never foretell what any one man will do, but you can say with precision what an average number will be up to. Individuals vary, but percentages remain constant.
Sherlock Holmes *in The Sign of Four.*

It is important to note that this system has been developed for Clinical Practice Guidelines. However, most of the underlying considerations regarding guidelines can also be applied as a framework for a structured reflection of primary information resources.

Categorizing the data as having a "high grade of evidence" means that you are very confident about the evidence. In reality, this grade is likely to be rather uncommon. Few medical "truths" can be expected to completely survive all future experimentation. After having decided on the graded quality of the evidence, the next step is to apply it to your patient's specific situation and requirements, i.e. the final step (Step 4) in the EBM process.

1
2
3
4

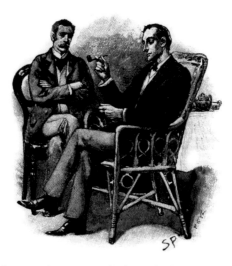

My dear Watson, you know my methods. Apply them.
Sherlock Holmes in *The Sign of Four.*

STEP 4
Employ the Results in Your Daily Practice

The final step in the EBM process is to *E*mploy the results (FIR*E*) in your practice. All patients request advice and recommendations for the management and treatment of their illness. A recommendation is based, however, on a complex framework of medical data, value systems and available resources. Each of these components needs to be tackled separately before a balanced recommendation can be presented to your patient. The further process of formulating a recommendation from your appraised studies includes several considerations:

- How generalizable are the results of the study?
- What is the expected balance between benefit and harm?
- What is the strength of the recommendation?
- What does your patient think?
- What is your recommendation?
- How do you communicate the information?

Applicability

The applicability of a study (external validity or generalizability) refers to the extent to which the results of a particular study can be used with patients other than the ones included in the study. Questions to ask in order to decide if the results of a study are applicable or not include the following:

- Are the results of this study appropriate for my patient?
- Could my patient have been included in this study? (Does my patient meet the inclusion and exclusion criteria used in this study?)
- Is there any reason to believe that the results presented would not apply to my patient?
- Does the study cover all clinically important aspects?
- Do the treatment benefits outweigh the potential harm and costs?

The institution that conducted the study may be specialized in the disease in question and perhaps the results presented (e.g. surgical complications) cannot be expected to apply in the care of your patient.

Efficacy is a measure of the effect of an intervention conducted under ideal or optimal conditions. *Effectiveness* denotes the results that can be obtained under normal conditions in a routine care setting. And if clear differences do exist in the setting in which the study was undertaken, is there a compelling reason to expect important differences in the size of the effect? Since most interventions have similar effects across most patient groups, you should not apply overly strict criteria when judging whether the results of a study are applicable to your patient. However, even if your patient appears to be perfectly similar to the patients in the study, you must take account of the fact that the results of treatment are not identical even in a homogeneous patient population. As a rule, there will be patients who respond very well to a treatment while others perhaps don't respond at all or may experience side-effects. Studies report mean values and their application to individual patients may yield other results than the expected ones.

Balance between benefit and harm

Before making a recommendation, you must consider whether or not the treatment benefits outweigh the potential harm and costs. To make this trade-off inevitably involves placing a relative value on the anticipated outcome(s).

It is often difficult to judge how much weight to give to different outcomes and different people will have different values. Most RCTs compare possible beneficial effects of one intervention with those of another. Therefore, issues related to harm often are not the main focus of RCTs or the trial may not include enough patients for unusual complications to occur. Most RCTs are powered to document benefitial effects, not to document complications. Systematic reviews/meta-analyses are preferably based on the results of RCTs and share the shortcomings of the included trials. In this respect, observational studies may offer an advantage for the documentation of harm.

Strength of Recommendation (SOR)

The strength of a recommendation refers to the probability that the application of a given recommendation will result in an improvement in health and it depends on the applicability of the evidence and the net benefits of an intervention. For the purpose of making recommendations more explicit, a number of different systems using either letters or numbers (or a combination of both) have been developed for the grading of a recommendation. One model [7] involves considerations of the quality of the evidence (p. 66), the applicability (p. 69) and the trade-off between benefit and harm.

Thus, the strength of a recommendation represents a weighted estimate of all anticipated positive and negative effects.

Strength of Recommendation (SOR)	Meaning
Net benefits	Good $>$ harm
Trade-offs	Good $=$ harm
Uncertain trade-offs	Good $\gtrless$ harm
No net benefits	Good $<$ harm

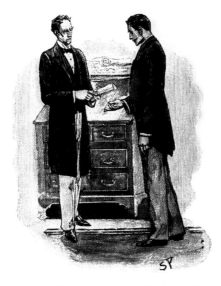

And I hope also that the cares of medical practise have not entirely obliterated the interest which you used to take in our little deductive problems.

Holmes to Watson in *The Stockbroker's Clerk.*

Patient's perceptions

The majority of published studies show "statistically significant" results. Regardless of whether a study has demonstrated statistically significant differences or not, it may have a degree of "clinical significance" that you are obliged to consider. Clinical significance implies that an attempt should be made to judge what the results would mean if they were applied to a population similar to the one studied. Useful calculations for assessing clinical significance are: the relative risk (RR), relative risk reduction (RRR), absolute risk reduction (ARR) and numbers needed-to-treat (NNT) (p. 46ff.).

The application of scientific data includes a discussion with your patient. What is the "personal significance" of the results, i.e. what does your patient think? The meaning of the concepts health and illness varies from individual to individual and the decision-making process is not necessarily either logical or rational. As Kant pointed out: "We do not look at things as they are, but as we are." Many patients value their present quality of life so highly that they hesitate to expose themselves to the risk of complications or to reduce the risk of symptoms which may appear much later. Patients with cancer have shown that they are prepared to accept massive chemotherapy to obtain a relatively small therapeutic benefit to a far greater extent than doctors and nurses are

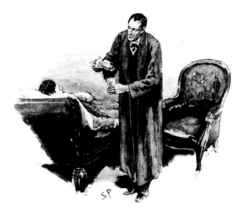

My dear fellow, said Sherlock Holmes as we sat in his lodgings at Baker Street, life is infinitely stranger than anything which the mind of man could invent.
Sherlock Holmes in *A case of Identity.*

prepared to do [11]. Certain patients would choose chemotherapy to live a week longer while others would refrain from chemotherapy even for a prolonged survival of two years [12].

Make a recommendation

Based on the strength of the recommendation and after having considered costs and explored patient values, a recommendation can be made [7]:

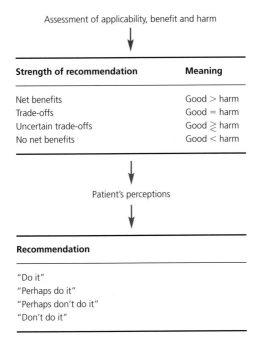

Assessment of applicability, benefit and harm

Strength of recommendation	Meaning
Net benefits	Good > harm
Trade-offs	Good = harm
Uncertain trade-offs	Good ≳ harm
No net benefits	Good < harm

Patient's perceptions

Recommendation
"Do it"
"Perhaps do it"
"Perhaps don't do it"
"Don't do it"

The recommendation to "Do it" or "Don't do it" indicates judgements that most well-informed patients would make. "Perhaps do it" or "Perhaps don't do it" indicate judgements that a majority of well-informed patients would make, but a substantial minority would not [7].

Communicating the evidence to your patient

The study results must be made understandable to the patient. In order to make it possible for the patient to reach an informed decision, medical data need to be translated into comprehensible information. The results of clinical trials are typically expressed as mean values but there are no such thing as an average patient in the real world. Your patient's participation can be obtained by a stepwise procedure [13]:

- Understand the patient's experience and expectations.
- Build a partnership.
- Provide evidence including a balanced discussion of uncertainties.
- Present recommendations based on clinical findings, the available scientific evidence and your patient's values.
- Check for understanding and seek agreement.

With this model, patients and their families can make an informed decision based on the available evidence and patient values.

Deduction, Analysis and Medicine

The key elements of Sherlock Holmes' strategy – the Science of Deduction and Analysis – have parallels with the diagnostic process employed in clinical medicine as well as with the process used when practicing EBM. Holmes stresses the importance of approaching a problem with a mind devoid of preconceived ideas or theories (*"Never guess. It is a shocking habit …"*) and of collection all facts before forming a hypothesis (*"… don't theorize before you have all the evidence."*). A good capacity for observation is also of great value according to Holmes (*"Observation with me is second nature."*) as is collecting all facts and recording all details, even those that are not immediately apparent (*"Your method should be founded upon the observation of trifles."*). The analogy to the EBM process consists in defining in detail the problem or carefully characterizing the patient and his/her disease state, what treatment options or diagnostic test you want to analyse and what outcome you are interested in, i.e., Step 1 (Formulate an Answerable Question) and Step 2 (Information Retrieval).

Holmes furthermore emphasizes the importance of collecting a large amount of information that is likely to result in the resolution of the problem (*"An investigator should look at everything."*) and then eliminate irrelevant facts (*"Whenever you have eliminated the impossible, whatever remains, however improbable, must be the truth."*). The EBM parallel to this is to initially ensure a high sensitivity in the search process and thereafter increase the specificity of the search.

The process of critical appraisal of the retrieved information (Step 3) is as demanding a task for health professionals as it is for detectives. In this respect, however, medicine has better tools at hand than the detective business has due to the availability of clinical epidemiology methods and formalized appraisal tools. The greatest challenge when practicing EBM, however, is its application to individual patients (Step 4) and, in this respect, there are no parallels to detective work.

If Sherlock Holmes had been a doctor today, would he stand out as being a superb one? No one can say for sure, but probably not. Even though his deductive skills would have been a great help, he would have probably had problems handling the large mass of available research evidence (*"… there comes a time when for every addition of knowledge you forget something that you knew before."*). He would probably have found that modern health care is more complex than any criminal case he handled as a detective. He might have also been surprised that the evidence base for the management of most diseases is still limited to this day. Not to mention the frustration that this fine detective would have experienced when confronted with patients with variable values and preferences. But the greatest frustration would have probably have come when he realized that medical problems can hardly ever be solved through a process of logic alone. It is therefore probable that today's medicine would offer little to keep him from returning to his familiar world of chemical flasks, magnifying glasses and fine tobaco [14].

By creating a "scientific detective" who could demonstrate the logical steps leading to his invariably correct conclusions, Conan Doyle gave the public a criminal catcher they could trust [15]. The use of EBM, however, will not invariably yield the optimal or best medical practice but it might increase the credibility of medicine and increase the prospect for more cost-effective and better care despite its limitations.

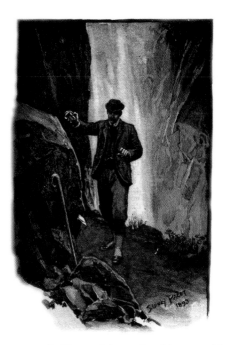

*Education never ends, Watson. It is a series of lessons with the greatest
for the last.*
Sherlock Holmes in *The Adventure of the Red Circle.*

References

1 Straus SE, et al. Evidence-Based Medicine. How to Practise and Teach EBM, 3rd edn. Churchill Livingstone, Edinburgh, 2005.

2 Hurwitz B. How does evidence-based guidance influence determinations of medical negligence? Br Med J 2004; 329:1024–8.

3 Shojania KG, Bero LA. Taking advantage of the explosion of systematic reviews: an efficient MEDLINE search strategy. Eff Clin Pract 2001; 4:157–62.

4 Hooper L, et al. Anti-oxidant foods or supplements for preventing cardiovascular disease (protocol for a Cochrane Review). Cochrane Library 2003; Issue 3.

5 Muin M, et al. SLIM: an alternative Web interface for MEDLINE/PubMed searches – a preliminary study. BMC Med Informat Decision Mak 2005, 5:37. www.biomedcentral.com/1472-6947/5/37

6 Vivekananthan DP, et al. Use of antioxidant vitamins for the prevention of cardiovascular disease: meta-analysis of randomised trials. Lancet 2003; 361:2017–23.

7 GRADE Working Group. Grading quality of evidence and strength of recommendations. Br Med J 2004; 328:1490–7.

8 Katrak P, et al. A systematic review of the content of critical appraisal tools. BMC Med Res Method 2004; 4:22.

9 Clarke M, Oxman AD. Cochrane Reviewer's Handbook 4.2.0. The Cochrane Collaboration, Oxford, 2003.

10 Premawardhena AP, et al. Low dose subcutaneous adrenaline to prevent acute adverse reactions to antivenom serum in people bitten by snakes: randomised, placebo controlled trial. Br Med J 1999; 318:1041–3.

11 Slevin ML, et al. Attitudes to chemotherapy: comparing views of patients with cancer with those of doctors, nurses and the general public. Br Med J 1990; 300:1458–60.

12 Silvestri G, et al. Preferences for chemotherapy in patients with advanced non-small cell lung cancer: descriptive study based on scripted interviews. Br Med J 1998; 317:771–5.

13 Epstein RM, et al. Communicating evidence for participatory decision making. J Am Med Assoc 2004; 291:2356–66.

14 Reed J. A medical perspective on the adventures of Sherlock Holmes. J Med Ethic Med Humanit 2001; 27:76–81.

15 Snyder LJ. Sherlock Holmes: Scientific Detective. Endeavour 2004; 28:104–8.

Summary of Information Sources and Search Engines

Secondary information sources (systematic reviews)

Database	Access via	Authorization
Cochrane Library	www.thecochranelibrary.com	Subscription; free in some countries
Clinical Queries	www.pubmed.gov	Free
Bandolier	www.jr2.ox.ac.uk/bandolier	Free
CRD databases	www.york.ac.uk/inst/crd	Free

Meta-search engines

Database	Access via	Authorization
TRIP Database	www.tripdatabase.com	Subscription
SUMSearch	http://sumsearch.uthscsa.edu	Free
Scirus	www.scirus.com	Free
Google	www.google.com	Free

Clinical Practice Guidelines

Database	Access via	Authorization
Clinical Evidence	www.clinicalevidence.com	Subscription
EBM Guidelines	www.ebm-guidelines.com	Subscription
FIRSTConsult	www.firstconsult.com	Subscription
NeLH	www.nelh.nhs.uk	Free
NICE	www.nice.org.uk	Free
PRODIGY	www.prodigy.nhs.uk	Free
NGC	www.guidelines.gov	Free
PIER	http://pier.acponline.org	Subscription
UptoDate	www.uptodate.com	Subscription

Primary information sources

Database	Access via	Authorization	Subject matter
MEDLINE			
PubMed:	www.pubmed.gov	Free	Medicine, bioscience,
OVID:	http://gateway.ovid.com	Subscription	education, health care
EMBASE	www.embase.com	Subscription	Medicine, pharmacology, nursing care
CINAHL	www.cinahl.com	Subscription	Physiotherapy, occupational therapy, nutrition
AMED	www.bl.uk; search: AMED	Subscription	Alternative medicine, physical therapy, occupational therapy, rehabilitation, palliative care
National Cancer Institute	www.cancer.gov	Free	Cancer
Psycinfo	www.apa.org/psycinfo	Subscription	Psychiatry, psychology

Internet-Based Spreadsheets

Organization	Accessible via	Spreadsheet
University of British Columbia	**www.healthcare.ubc.ca** (Go to Links then to Calculators)	Risk calculations, odds, sensivity, specificity, LR (Bayes)
Scottish Intercollegiate Guidelines Network	**www.sign.ac.uk** (Go then to Methodology and on to Risk Calculator)	Risk calculations, odds
Vassar College	**http://faculty.vassar.edu/ lowry/VassarStats.html** (Go to Clinical Research Calculators)	Risk calculations, odds
University of Toronto	**www.cebm.utoronto.ca/ Practise/ca/statscal**	Risk assessments, odds, sensitivity, specificity, LR (Bayes)
University of California	**www.stat.ucla.edu** (Go to Statistical Calculators)	Many different ones

Sherlock Holmes References

Doyle AC. The Complete Sherlock Holmes. Gramercy Books, New York, 2002.
www.sherlockian.net/resources/media.html
http://camdenhouse.ignisart.com/gallery/index.html

List of Illustrations

Sidney Paget's original illustrations have been used throughout.

The Adventures of Sherlock Holmes: The Red-headed League, p. 8; The Speckled Band, pp. xii, 41; The Engineer's Thumb, p. 72.

Memoris of Sherlock Holmes: Silver Blaze, p. 43; The Stockbroker's Clerk, p. 60; The Musgrave Rituals, pp. viii, 22; The Reigate Puzzle, p. 28; The Crooked Man, p. 18, 47, 77;
The Greek Interpreter, p. 68; The Naval Treaty, pp. 13, 34, 71; The Final Problem, pp. 18, 47, 77;

The Return of Sherlock Holmes: The Priorty School, p. 3; The Golden Pince-nez, pp. 37, 54; The Missing Three-quarters, p. 52; The Abbey Grange, pp. 10, 15, 50.

All cover illustrations taken from **Memoirs of Sherlock Holmes**: The Reigate Puzzle, The Final Problem, The Musgrave Ritual and The Naval Treaty.

Recommended EBM Literature

- Ajetunmobi O. Making Sense of Critical Appraisal. Arnold, London, 2002.
- Black ER, Bordley DR, Tape TG, Panzer RJ. Diagnostic Strategies for Common Medical Problems. American College of Physicians, Philadelphia, 1999.
- Fletcher RW, Fletcher SW. Clinical Epidemiology. The Essentials, 4th ed. Lippincott Williams & Wilkins, Baltimore, 2005.
- Greenhalgh T. How to Read a Paper: The Basics of Evidence-based Medicine. Blackwell Publishing (BMJ Books imprint), Oxford, 2006.
- Guyatt G, Drummond R. User's Guides to the Medical Literature. American Medical Association (AMA) Press, Chicago, 2002.
- Heneghan C, Badenhoch D. Evidence-based Medicine Toolkit, 2nd edition. Blackwell Publishing (BMJ Books imprint), Oxford, 2006.

Glossary

Absolute risk reduction (ARR): Difference between an event in the control group and an event in the experimental group.

Allocation concealment: A method of generating a sequence that ensures random allocation between two or three arms of a study, without revealing this to either study subjects or researchers.

Applicability (see Validity, external): The ability to generalize the results of one study to a larger population of similar patients.

Bias: A factor that influences the results of an investigation above and beyond the experimental intervention.

Blinding: Study participants and observers are kept ignorant of the group to which the subjects are assigned.

Boolean operators (named after George Boole): The search terms AND, OR and NOT are used during literature searches to include or exclude certain citations from electronic databases.

Case–control study: A study in which patients with a certain outcome are compared with patients not having this outcome and in which one looks for factors that might cause the differences between the groups.

Case report: A report on individual patients.

Clinical Practice Guideline: A recommendation elaborated with due consideration of evidence-based principles and intended to provide scientific support for decisions on the treatment of specific disease entities or other health care matters.

Coefficient of variation (CV): The standard deviation expressed as a percentage of the mean. $CV = (SD/mean) \times 100$.

Cohort: A group of patients having a number of characteristics in common.

Cohort study: An observational study in which the individuals are grouped according to their previously being exposed, or *not* exposed, to some type of phenomenon and are then followed over time.

Confidence interval (CI): The spread of the results of a study within which the true value is expected to lie.

Confounder: A factor that interferes with the variable being studied by virtue of the fact that it is related in some way to the outcome under study.

Consecutive-case study: A number of patients with the same outcome are studied without a control group.

Cross-sectional study: Observations concerning a defined group of patients are made at a specific point in time (or time interval).

Effectiveness: The extent to which a specific intervention produces a beneficial outcome in the routine setting.

Efficacy: The extent to which a specific intervention produces a beneficial outcome under ideal conditions.

External validity: See Validity.

False-negative result: No effect has been found although, in reality, there is one.

False-positive result: An effect has been found although, in reality, there is not one.

Generalizability: see Applicability

Impact factor (IF): A parameter of the frequency with which the articles of a certain journal are referred to in those of other journals.

Intention-to-treat: The results for all individuals initially recruited are included in the final compilation of results. The results for individuals who, for one reason or another, did not complete the study are also included in the compilation of results.

Internal validity: See Validity.

MeSH (Medical Subject Headings): Indexing and classification system within MEDLINE consisting of specific subject headings describing the contents of articles.

Meta-analysis: A systematic review in which quantitative methods are used to compile the results from separate, but similar, comparable studies (usually RCT).

Numbers-needed-to-treat (NNT): Number of patients that must be treated for an effect to occur in one patient; NNT = 1/ARR.

Numbers-needed-to-harm (NNH): Number of patients treated for whom there is one additional patient who experiences an episode of harm (adverse effect, complication, etc.). It is calculated in the same manner as NNT.

Odds: The ratio between two probabilities – the probability of an event to that of a non-event.

Odds ratio (OR): The odds for an experiment group showing positive or, conversely, negative effects of an intervention in relation to a control group.

Outcome: The measurable result of an effect on the health or condition of a patient or population.

Post-test probability: Proportion of patients with a positive test result that have the disease.

Power: The probability that a test will give rise to a significant difference at a certain level of significance.

Prevalence: The fundamental risk of a disease occurring in the population in question.

Pre-test probability: See Prevalence.

Probability: The proportion of patients in whom a particular characteristic is present.

***p*-value:** The possibility of a certain event being due to chance.

Randomized-controlled trial (RCT): A study in which a group of patients are allocated to either an experiment or control group.

Relative risk (RR): The ratio of the risk of an event occurring in the experimental group to the risk of it occurring in the control group.

Relative risk reduction (RRR): The percentage reduction of events occurring in the experiment group compared with those in the control group.

Reliability: The degree of stability of a test to produce the same result if the measurement is repeated under identical conditions.

Reproducibility: The extent to which the results are identical, or nearly identical, every time the test is repeated.

Secondary information source: A compilation of original data vetted for quality.

Sensitivity, of a diagnostic test: The proportion of patients with a disease showing a positive test result.

Sensitivity, of an information search: Expresses the ability to find all relevant articles in a search.

Specificity, of a diagnostic test: The proportion of patients not having a disease and showing a negative test result.

Specificity, of an information search: Expresses the ability to exclude irrelevant articles in a search.

Surrogate measurement: Use of a measuring method which in and of itself is not clinically important but is related in some way to a clinically important effect.

Systematic review: A report in the making of which independent reviewers have systematically searched, critically examined and summarized the whole body of medical literature on a specific subject.

Type I error (alpha error): A study finds a difference when no such difference actually exists.

Type II error (beta error): A study fails to find a difference when such a difference actually exists.

Validity: The extent to which a test method measures what it is intended to measure. Its **internal validity** refers to the experimental design of the study itself for measuring what is intended to be measured. Its **external validity** refers to the extent to which the results of the study can be used on other patients than the ones included in the study.

Index

Note: Page numbers in *italics* refer to tables.

absolute risk reduction, 47–48, 72
ACP Journal Club, 17, 44
    appraisal protocol, for diagnostic
        studies, 58
AGREE, 43
AHRQ (Agency for Healthcare
        Research and Quality), 17
alpha error, *see* type I error
allocation concealment, 46
applicability, 69–70
    see also generalizability; validity

Bandolier, 7
beta error, *see* type II error
blinding, 46
Boolean search, 21

case-control study, 39
case report, 39
Centre for Reviews and Dissemination
        (CRD) databases, 8
Clinical Evidence, 11
Clinical Practice Guidelines, *13*
    Clinical Evidence, 11
    critical appraisal, 64–65
    EBM Guidelines, 11
    FIRSTConsult, 11
    NeLH, 11–12
    NGC, 12
    NICE, 12

    PIER, 12
    PRODIGY, 12
Clinical Queries, in PubMed, 7
Cochrane Library
    databases, 6–7, 16
Cochrane Reviews (Cochrane Database
        of Systematic Reviews), 6
coefficient of variation, 59
cohort study, 39
confidence interval (CI), 49
CONSORT, 42
critical appraisal
    of Clinical Practice Guidelines, 64–65
    of diagnostic studies, 51–60
    of systematic review/meta-analysis,
        60–64
    of therapy studies, 44–51
critical appraisal tool, 42
    key items, for quality assessment,
        42–43
Critically Appraised Topics (CATs), 5, 14
cross-sectional study, 39

database search strategy, in PubMed
    Details function, 22–23
    History function, 23–24
    Limits function, 28

EBM Clinical Practice Guidelines, 11
EBM Online, 16–17

EBM portals
  ACP Journal Club, 17, 44, 58
  AHRQ, 17
  EBM Online, 16–17
  INAHTA, 16
  netting the evidence, 17
  NLM, 14, 16
effectiveness, 70
efficacy, 70
EMBASE, 14
Employ results, in EBM process
  applicability, 69–70
  benefit and harm, balance, 70
  communicating evidence, to
      patients, 73–74
  patient's perceptions, 72–73
  strength of recommendation, for
      patients, 70–71, 73
external validity, 35, 51
  see applicability; generalizability;
      validity

FIRE approach in EBM, xii, 1, 19, 35, 69
FIRSTConsult, 11
free textword searches, 20

generalizability, *see* applicability;
      external validity
Google, 9–10

Hierarchy of Evidence, *38*

impact factor, 40–41, *40*
INAHTA (International Network of
      Agencies for Health Technology
      Assessment), 16
information resources, 4
  CATs, 5, 14
  Clinical Practice Guidelines, 11–13,
      64–65
  database selection, 5
  library resources, 16
  meta-search engines, 9–10
  primary information sources, 14–15

systematic reviews, 4–5, 5–8
information search
  database search strategy, in PubMed,
      22–24, 28
  procedure, in PubMed, 19
intention-to-treat, 45
internal validity, 35
  see also validity
internet-based spreadsheets, *81*

Level of Evidence, grading, 39
library resources
  university libraries, 16
likelihood ratio, 51, 57–58
  for negative test result (LR−),
      55, 57
  for positive test result (LR+),
      55–57

Medical Subject Headings (MeSH)
      terms, 20–21, 26–27, *30*
MEDLINE, 7, 14, 16, 20
meta-analysis, 4–7, 60–64
meta-search engines, 5, 9–10, *10*
  Google, 9–10
  Scirus, 9
  SUMSearch, 9
  TRIP, 9, 20

National Library of Medicine (NLM),
      14, 16
NeLH (National Electronic Library for
      Health), 11–12
netting the evidence, 17
NGC (National Guideline
      Clearinghouse), 12
NICE (National Institute for Health
      and Clinical Excellence), 12
numbers-needed-to-treat, 46–49, 72
numbers-needed-to-harm, 49

odds, 47–48, 51–52
odds ratio (OR), 47–48, 61
OVID, 14, *15*, 16

PICO approach, in EBM, 1–2
PIER (Physician's Information and
       Education Resource), 12
predictive value, 51, 54–56
prevalence, 55–58
primary information sources, *15*
    EMBASE, 14
    PubMed, 7, 14, 20
probability, 51–52
PRODIGY, 12
PubMed, 7, 14, *15*, 20
    Search procedure, 19–24, 27–33
    Clinical Queries, 7
p-value, 49

quality assessment, of information, 35
    critical appraisal, study types of, 43
    grading
        Level of Evidence, 39
        quality of evidence, 66–67
        study design analysis, 36–41
quality of evidence, grading, 66–67
question formulation, for evidence-
       based medicine (EBM)
    information resources, 4
    PICO approach, 1–2
QUORUM, 42

randomized control trial (RCT), 28, 30,
       35, 37–40, 44, 70
Related Articles function, 32–33
relative risk, 47–48, 72
reliability, 35–36
reproducibility, 59

Science of Deduction and Analysis, 75
scientific quality evaluation, 41
    critical appraisal
        of Clinical Practice Guidelines,
            64–65
        of diagnostic studies, 51–60
        of systematic review/meta-
            analysis, 60–64
        of therapy studies, 44–51

Scirus, 9
search results, restricting, 27
    Limits function, 28
secondary information sources,
       see systematic reviews
sensitivity
    of diagnostic test, 54–58
    of information search, 20–21
SLIM (Slider Interface for MEDLINE/
       PubMed searches), 29
specificity
    of diagnostic test, 51, 54–56
    of information search, 27–30
STARD (Standard for Reporting of
       Diagnostic Accuracy), 42
Strength of Recommendation, 70, *71*, 73
study design analysis
    experimental studies, 37
    observational studies, 37–39
    randomized-controlled trial
        (RCT), 38
SUMSearch, 9
surrogate parameter, 65
Systematic reviews, 4–5, *5*, *8*
    Bandolier, 7
    Clinical Queries, in PubMed, 7
    Cochrane Library, 6–7
    CRD databases, 8
    critical appraisal of, 60–64

Technology Assessments database, 7
TRIP (Turning Research into Practice
       Database), 9, 20
type I error, 50
type II error, 50

UptoDate, 13

validity, 35–36

wide information search, in PubMed
    Boolean search, 21
    free textword searches, 20
    with MeSH terms, 20–21